Overcoming Stress and Anxiety

A Simple Guide for Understanding and Reducing Stress and Anxiousness

Alex Bruce

Copyright © 2022 Alex Bruce
All rights reserved.
ISBN-13:979-8-8407-4622-6

To Andrew

Contents

Introduction

Mindfully choosing to take the step to cure ourselves, is mindfully choosing to take the step to cure the world.

Stress-related conditions, including anxiety, are currently the #1 reason for doctor visits in North America. It is normal to feel besieged at times with stressful or anxious thoughts, feelings and emotions. In fact, it is normal to feel stressed or anxious even by reading, thinking, or talking about these things.

Knowing that you are normal, that what you are experiencing is typical, and that you will be okay, are the first steps in transforming your relationship to stress or anxiety.

That being said, although it is normal for all of us who are humanizing on this planet to be stressed or anxious at times, it is not optimal. The good thing is that there is much that can be done to help you to think, feel and live differently.

There are two very common beliefs that we experience when we feel as though we are swimming (or drowning) in stress or anxiety:

#1) That we are the only one who feels this way

#2) That things can/will never change

Thankfully, both of those beliefs are undeniably untrue. Suffering from stress or anxiety does not have to be your reality. Just because that's the way something has always been, doesn't mean that that's the way it will always be. Although it is clearly not possible to completely eradicate stress or anxiety from our lives, as they are both a normal part of being human, it is possible to learn how to create a new relationship with your emotions; one that is mindful and compassionate. There is hope, and you are closer to feeling better than you think.

Sometimes the smallest comment, or the tiniest piece of knowledge can blow our mind – forever changing our way of thinking, living or being, in a deeply and profoundly meaningful way. It is my deepest hope that you will find that here.

Over the years, I have educated people about stress and anxiety reduction in all types of schools, programs, organizations and workplaces, and these tools are all incredibly versatile; many of them supportive whether a person is 5 years old or 105. In changing a relationship with stress or anxiety, we don't just want a toolbox, we want a *robust* toolbox, and as such, I invite you to give these practices a try and find out what works for you. We do not have fire drill practices in the middle of a fire – we have them when things are safe so that we can think rationally, and practice what to do in the event of a fire so that we have the process memorized should a fire ever break out. Just like practicing fire drills, when you practice these tools, these different ways of living or of viewing life, they will be readily available for you when and if you need them so that stress or anxiety no longer have the power to overwhelm you.

As this guide is packed full with hundreds of quick tips, mindful exercises, tools and techniques for moving your physiology past dysregulation and transforming your relationship with stress and anxiety, I also invite you to really mark this book up; you may find that dog-earring the pages or underlining, highlighting, or circling different sections will facilitate finding details that were of significance or resonance for you if you are ever in need of the information in a hurry. Moving through the pages of this simple guide we will investigate the who, the what, the where, the when, and the why of stress and anxiety. Most importantly, throughout this book we will cover a multitude of techniques for the *how's* - how to befriend feeling anxious or stressed and how to overcome these feelings, including the most crucial "how" of all...

"Over every mountain there is a path, though it may not be seen from the valley."

– Theodore Roethke

One thing to remember is that you are an incredibly unique individual; quite literally one of a kind. Like a sudoku puzzle with only one combination of numbers that work, there is a combination of tools and techniques that will be the perfect match for you. Just as you may likely try on several pairs of shoes before finding the perfect fit, please be open and curious as you discover exactly what *you* need to know, try, or do in order to optimize your mental health and wellbeing!

Part I: The Who

Experiencing stress or anxiety is not pleasant. In fact, it can be quite awful. At times, it can feel overwhelming, paralyzing, all-encompassing, and suffocating. Either one of them can be embarrassing to say the least and downright debilitating or life-limiting to say the worst. Not only that, but adding to the pain and excruciation is that these emotions can feel very isolating. Sadly, they are often a scary and lonely place to be.

So, here's the truth: You are not alone. The "Who" of anxiety is inclusive of pretty much every single human being on the planet. Frankly, it can include animals as well – my beloved cat used to lose the fur around his little kitty face whenever I had to travel. The point is that although these stressful states try to get us to believe that we are alone in feeling these feelings, emoting these emotions and thinking anxious thoughts, we are not. And as much as they try to convince us that we are "lesser" than others, we are not. These thoughts and beliefs are simply tricks that stress and anxiety play on us to keep us in their grasp.

Mindful Reminder: *Stress and anxiety are physiological states, not character flaws!*

Who exactly is the "who" of anxiety or stress? It is you, it is me, and it includes the billions of other human beings that are alive on this planet now, have been alive in the past, and will be alive in the future. Feeling stressed or anxious is a part of being human, but it isn't the only part of being human, and doesn't even have to be a large part of our experience. Included in these pages are the tools you will need to liberate yourself from being stuck in stressful states.

"Vulnerability in the face of constant change is what we share, whatever our present condition."

– Sharon Salzberg

Gentle Reminder: *The "who" of anxiety is all of us. You are not alone.*

As we will discuss and discover, stress and anxiety are merely tools that our minds and bodies use to communicate with us; we simply need to learn how to read and use them. But rarely can we ever solve these issues using the same psychology that got us into them in the first place, so if you are someone who has a tendency to be hard on yourself, possibly someone who learned to be "tough" earlier on in life in order to survive, or was not brought up in a home where you learned to offer yourself care and tenderness, now is the time to invite a change to your perspective and to begin your journey from a new starting point. Being kind to oneself is truly a game-changer – a superpower, and it is something that is accessible to all of us with practice.

Mindful Tip: *Instead of thinking, "…my anxiety" or, "I'm stressed", considering simply recognizing, "Oh, anxiety is present" or, "Look at that, stress just arrived on the scene." As a replacement for viewing them as a curse, curiously investigate if you can view stress or anxiety as a gift; a gateway to new openings and learnings that you are soon to discover. As impossible as it may seem right now, living life with a gentle sense of curiosity and self-inquiry can be like having a love-affair with your experience of being human*

Mindful Exercise: Self-Compassion

Feeling as though we are isolated in our stressful states only serves to create more feelings of isolation and anxiety. Instead, choose to take another step towards feeling better: Self-compassion. Leading expert in self-compassion and author of many books, including *Self-Compassion: The Proven Power of Being Kind to Yourself,* Dr.

Kristin Neff tells us that self-compassion includes three important components:

1) Recognize that you are experiencing a moment of suffering
2) Acknowledge that you are a part of humanity, and that at times, all of humanity has moments of suffering like this
3) Offer yourself some compassion, much like the compassion that you would wish to receive from a loving friend or caregiver

The exercise may look something like this:

1) "Wow, anxiety sucks. This is really hard, and I wish I didn't have these anxious thoughts and feelings."

   * Find language that fits for you, and allow yourself to really sink into the acknowledgement of your suffering

2) "Everyone feels like this sometimes. I am not alone. I am connected to everyone because everyone experiences anxiety in their life – this is part of being human."

   * Again, use language that lands for you, and invite yourself to truly *connect* to the fact that you are humanly human, just like all other human beings on the planet

3) "You can get through this. You have made it through other tough times and you can do this, too. Things will get better and everything will be okay."

* Don't force anything here, encourage yourself with self-kindness that resonates for you. If self-compassion is difficult for you, then even *wishing* to be more self-compassionate with yourself is an act of self-compassion and should be considered a win. What would you say to someone that you dearly loved who was going through the same thing?

<u>Mindful Tip:</u> *Any type of sympathetic mobilization (including anxiety or stress) can create inflammation in the body. When inflammation occurs, it can lower our stress and anxiety thresholds, making us more prone to stress and anxiety, which then increases our levels of inflammation – without intervention, the cycle can continue. People who regularly practice self-compassion get over stress and anxiety faster than those who don't. Although it is typical for people who struggle with stress or anxiety to resist being self-compassionate, for fear that it will make them 'lazy' or 'weak', these myths have been clinically researched and determined to be untrue. For many reasons, actively taking steps of self-care, self-love and self-compassion are <u>necessary ingredients</u> in overall health and wellness*

<u>Quick Tip:</u> *Go easy on yourself; give yourself a break – it's healthier for you that you can even imagine!*

"All of us might wish at times that we lived in a more tranquil world, but we don't. And if our

times are difficult and perplexing, so are they challenging and filled with opportunity."

– Robert Kennedy

Part II: The What

What exactly even *is* anxiety? What *is* stress? We can't see them, but we can see what happens when we or others suffer with them. We can't touch them, but we know all too well what they feel like. We can't hear them coming, but we all know what they sound like, and we can't smell or taste them, but they do indeed exist. So, what are they then?

Basically, stress and anxiety are overactivations of our nervous system that our current circumstances don't require.

That's it.

Sometimes we experience stress or anxiety in the body, such as tightness or shaking, sometimes we experience them in our mind with racing, ruminating or depressive thoughts, and sometimes we experience them in our emotions.

Different from fear, which alerts us to an immediate risk requiring immediate action, stress and anxiety do not represent an immediate risk. Where fear can be helpful and necessary, anxiety is not helpful nor necessary (even though it tries to convince us that it is both). For example, if we are about to walk across the street and a car runs a red light, careening towards us, we would experience fear. Within a fraction of a second, our brain alerts our body to secrete stress hormones that propel us into action in order to flee. The alarm centre of our brain takes over, rendering rational thought helpless, and we immediately move into safety, jumping out of the way of the car. That was fear doing what it was supposed to do; moving us into action to either fight, freeze, or in this scenario, flee.

However, anxiety is all about living in fear of something that *may or may not happen in the future.* Where actual fear often indicates something concretely imminent, stress and anxiety often represent something imagined. In fact, for most of us on the planet, anxiety is about living in imagined fear of something that is quite likely *never* going to happen in the future.

Mindful Reminder: *If something truly was a "life or death" situation, the resulting experience would be fear not anxiety*

Regrettably, both stress and anxiety create a similar bodily response as fear – our brain detects a threat and sends out those reactionary hormones and chemicals in order to propel us into action. However, there is often nowhere to go, so we just steep ourselves in chemical soup. This chemical-soup steeping can lead us to physical and/or mental illness, which further exacerbates our feelings of stress. It can, and often does become a self-perpetuating cycle of feeling anxious.

The excellent news is that there are a host of things that we can do to stop this cycle in its tracks and we each just need to find the right combination of tools that work for us as individuals. What works for some may not work for others and vice versa, so I encourage you to give them all a try and see what fits.

Mindful Reminder: *People often believe that if only they could figure out what was making them anxious that they wouldn't be anxious anymore. How effective has that been? Remember that the body doesn't just need thoughts, it needs regulation…breathe and relax in order to communicate to your body that it is safe.*

Mindful Exercise: Be Here Now

One of the many ways that we stress ourselves out is through the process of rumination; getting stuck in a cycle of unhelpful and anxious thoughts. These thoughts are generally focussed on an event or events that might happen in the future or an event or events that happened in the past and that we wish had been different. Basically, rumination is simply a form of time travelling; wherever our mind may go when we ruminate – to the past or the future - it is not in the present moment.

Research clearly indicates that the happiest and healthiest people in the world are the ones who can stay in the present moment. This very moment right now, without any mind wandering. That means that for the most part, we would be well-served to not get stuck in ruminating about the past or worrying about the future. How do we do that? We be here now. If it feels comfortable for you, give it a try as you read along. (If you would like to close your eyes, you may wish to record the instructions on your phone, speaking slowly as you read, and pausing in between each point in order to provide yourself with time to experience the exercise.)

Be Here Now

When you find that your mind has been hijacked with intrusive thoughts, take these steps:

1) Recognize that you are having thoughts that are not based in the present moment.

    *There is no need to beat yourself up or berate yourself for anything here, just non-judgementally acknowledge, "Oh, look at that – my mind has taken off again." There is no shame here, we all do it.

2) Slowly and kindly say to yourself, either silently or aloud, "Be here now."

3) Bring yourself back to the present moment. This can be done through myriad ways, including taking a long, slow, deep breath or connecting to a part of your body such as the sensation of your sit bones being supported by a chair, your feet on the ground, or your hands resting on your lap. You may also choose to place your awareness on sounds, such as

the birds chirping outside your window, or the air conditioning unit in the building. Perhaps you would prefer to connect to what you are seeing – really investigating the look of a table that you are near – is it shiny or dull, smooth or bumpy, patterned or plain, etc., or looking for different items in your vicinity that are the color green (or blue, or yellow, or grey...)

> * The point here is to interrupt the intrusive thought patterns by finding something that is comfortable for you to focus on that is in the "now". If you focus on something that perpetuates your stress levels (such as noticing that your breathing is shallow or that your hands are shaking), then simply find something that is neutral for you. Once again, this is not a one-size-fits-all solution; it's a buffet where you get to figure out what you and your body are in the mood for at this point in time.

4) Slowly and softly say or think to yourself again, "Be here now." Let the statement truly sink in. Recognize that intrusive or ruminating thoughts are not a realistic representation of what is happening in this present moment. Continue to connect with the fact that you are here, in this moment, by bringing your mind to meet your body or surroundings.

5) If it is helpful, you may want to repeat to yourself, "You are not there. You are here. Be here now." Repeat as necessary.

As with all of the mindful exercises that we will cover in this guide, this becomes easier and more accessible with regular practice. This is a tool that you may choose to use when you are already feeling anxious, or merely notice that your mind has wandered off while you are doing your grocery shopping, work, or listening to someone speak.

Free Resource: *A wonderful combination of both levity and authentic presence can be found in Dr. Darry Tonemah's podcast "The Singing Psychologist"*

If you prefer, here is an alternative to Be Here Now:

Mindful Exercise: I am Aware

1) Recognize that your mind has wandered

2) Say or think softly to yourself, "I am aware"

3) Open your awareness to any or all of your senses. While breathing slowly and deeply, become more aware: What else can you hear when you expand your sense of sound? What else can you see if you open and increase your frontal and peripheral vision? What can you smell? What taste do you have in your

mouth? What can you sense your body touching (such as hands on the steering wheel, or the sensation of holding a pen or standing on the ground)?

4) Repeat as necessary, slowly and softly, "I am aware." Connect with your awareness in the present moment as if it is an expanding bubble of sights and sensations.

Both of those mindful exercises are to support our nervous systems in finding a calmer state. So often, we try to *think* ourselves into feeling better, but it can be very difficult and counterproductive to do that. Not only is it challenging to collect our thoughts when we are in a heightened state of stress or anxiety, but the attempts to *control* our thoughts and *make* them less anxious can often lead to more anxiety. Instead, it is often more beneficial for us to *feel* ourselves into feeling better. This includes a relaxed body, slow, deep, calm breathing and the awareness of the fact that in this moment, you are safe. This helps to settle the mind, and when our mind and body reach this state, we no longer feel anxious.

Mindful Tip: *Thoughts such as, "There is no reason for me to be feeling this way!" or "Only losers get stressed and anxious; I should be stronger/ better than this!" are full of blame, guilt, and shame, which only work to exacerbate levels of activation. Do you know who doesn't get stressed or anxious? Psychopaths or fakers. You are okay. We can even self-shame and create stress and* *anxiety around not feeling a certain way, "Why am I not excited? Why am I jealous of someone that I care about? Why am I scared of making a positive change, such as leaving a toxic relationship or job?" Any change – good or bad – can create stress or anxiety. Offer some softness to yourself. Try replacing self-deprecating thoughts with self-compassion; "It sure is hard being human, and we all go through times like this. How can I support myself best in this moment?"*

Part III: The Where

In order to understand where anxiety comes from, we will need to take a little journey to the brain, investigating two parts in particular:

The first part of the brain that we will investigate is commonly referred to as the amygdala (there are actually two of them in the brain, plural form "amygdalae") which works as the smoke detector of the brain. It is the part of the brain that we inherited from our lizard friends that is responsible for fight, flight, freeze and faint. When the amygdala "smells smoke" (detects a possible threat) it will engage the nervous system and mobilize the fight/flight response, for which we will use the analogy of the internal sprinkler system. If the amygdala detects a threat (smells smoke), it will immediately engage the sympathetic nervous system (the sprinklers) in order to keep the body safe (put out the fire). This works perfectly if there actually *is* a fire, such as if you were faced with debris flying out of a window toward you and you quickly needed to duck (flee) to safety. The amygdala is responsible for threat elimination. The amygdala is *not* responsible for sophisticated thought processes including memory, future consideration, connection with others, or even conscious thought, which is why when we have been triggered, we often say or do things that we later regret. (The amygdala is often – albeit not always - the culprit behind decisions that are impulsive, short-sighted, narcissistic, and self-centered or self-serving.) Basically, the rational part of our brain was "turned off" as the amygdala did its version of keeping us safe. Regrettably, this might look something like making a rude gesture out the window if someone cuts you off in traffic (fight response), hanging up the phone if someone says something that you don't agree with (flight response), or drawing a complete blank when you come face to face with a test paper (freeze response). The amygdala can be an absolute life-saver when dealing with actual danger or life-threat, but can create some "not-your-best-moments" when the danger it perceived wasn't an actual threat.

The good news is that we have another part of our brain known as the pre-frontal cortex (PFC for short) that is akin to the calm and resourceful firefighter. When the smoke alarm goes off (the amygdala) then we want to get the firefighter there as soon as possible so that they can assess the situation. If it was indeed a fire, then the sprinkler system (sympathetic nervous system) would have doused it. If not, we will want to turn the sprinklers off quickly (calm the nervous system) so that there isn't any fallout from the damage that may have occurred.

The amygdala is the "where" of stress and anxiety and the pre-frontal cortex is the "where" of rational and compassionate thought. (Of course, there are other elements of the brain that come into play here, but for the purposes of keeping it simple, we'll stick with these two major players.) Sadly, most of us didn't learn how to train our internal firefighter to respond quickly when we were little, which is why so many of us struggle with keeping anxiety, anger, stress, and depression at bay. Happily, we know a lot more now than we ever have, and (thanks to brain plasticity) can quite simply "train" our PFC to respond faster. Anytime that we notice that the alarm of the amygdala has been triggered (which we will investigate further in subsequent pages), we can use mindful awareness to notice that we've been activated and then *choose* to engage the PFC. Practicing any or all of the Mindful Exercises in this guide will help.

> **Mindful Tip:** *Remember that anything that is happening in your body is simply information. You do not have to label it as anything other than that, and you do not have to view it as distressing*

Mindful Exercise: Name It to Tame It

Dr. Dan Siegel is a Clinical Professor of Psychiatry at the UCLA School of Medicine and author of many books including *Aware: The Science and Practice of Presence.* Dr. Siegel has popularized the term "Name It to Tame It" in order to support people in bringing their PFC back online after the amygdala has been triggered.

Anytime you notice that you are stressed or anxious, that indicates that the amygdala has been activated. This can be because of an actual threat, or simply a ringing phone on a busy day, some unsupportive or self-critical self-talk, or an upcoming weigh-in or blood pressure monitoring with your doctor. It's important to get the PFC activated in order to take over so that you don't do anything you might later regret (such as be anxious unnecessarily). We can "force" the pre-frontal cortex back on-line (taking back control of the brain) by consciously choosing to engage in rational thought. As the amygdala doesn't think rationally, it has to cool down and back away in order for the PFC to take over. Simply naming what you are experiencing (which requires rational thought, sensory attention, communication skills, etc.) forces the pre-frontal cortex region of the brain to take over. When we "see" the emotion, we don't have to "be" the emotion, and when resistance dissolves, things get easier. Hence, using the PFC to "name" what is happening for you works to "tame" the amygdala.

- Sitting or standing where you are, eyes open or closed, become aware of your emotional state – are you tired, or hungry, or jealous about something, or happy, or angry, or calm, or curious…? Without judgement, just investigate the emotion or emotions that are present for you. Some of the emotions may even contradict one another, or be emotions that you would rather not admit that you have – let go of any shoulding or repressing; it is okay to be human. Really connect to how you authentically feel in a kind, self-compassionate, and inquisitive manner.

- Now become aware of your physical sensations. Is your chest tight or relaxed? Is your stomach calm or relaxed? Are you muscles soft or tense? What sensations do you have in your body? Again, this is simply a gentle inquiry, a loving curiosity into how you are feeling physically without the need to create any stories.

- Take a deep breath and connect with how you feel versus a moment ago before this exercise

Mindful Tip: *Don't feel like naming it? Consider drawing how you feel instead*

Poem: The Guest House

This being human is a guest house.

Every morning a new arrival

A joy, a depression, a meanness,

some momentary awareness comes

as an unexpected visitor.

Welcome and entertain them all!

Even if they are a crowd of sorrows,

who violently sweep your house

empty of its furniture,

still, treat each guest honorably.

He may be clearing you out

for some new delight.

The dark thought, the shame, the malice.

meet them at the door laughing and invite them in.

Be grateful for whatever comes.

because each has been sent

as a guide from beyond.

—Rumi, translation by Coleman Barks

Mindful Tip: *Having an extensive emotional vocabulary is incredibly supportive for reducing stress and anxiety, as not knowing what an emotion is, or which emotion one is feeling, can often be a breeding ground for heightened dysregulation. ("I don't know what's wrong with me!") If you feel that you could use a brush-up with your emotional fluency, there are card decks, emojis and charts to help with this. If you prefer, simply google "list of emotions." And know that one of the large causes of stress or anxiety can be grief; grief that something did or did not happen, something that changed or stopped or ended. It is okay to provide* *yourself with support (or to get some) in order to move through grief – like it or not, it is yet another path in the journey of being human*

Free Resource: *To check out Dan Siegel's blogs, access them at: www.drdansiegel.com. You may want to also try out his "Wheel of Awareness" meditation on YouTube. For people who are newer to meditation, I suggest the 25-minute version versus the seven-minute version, which can be challenging to keep up with.*

Part IV: The When

The "When" of stress or anxiety is anytime the amygdala has sensed a threat. As each of us are wired differently, it means that we are all programmed to sense threat in varying ways. This is a perfect example of where self-reflection plays a pivotal role in your journey to befriend and overcome anxiety: Identifying sources of stress and anxiety is a crucial step in managing them.

When are the times when your anxiety is most heightened? Perhaps it is at night, when the room is dark and quiet and you are left only with the thoughts that you have been trying to avoid all day. Maybe your stress arrives when you have to make a presentation to your manager or approach an unapproachable co-worker for help. Possibly they occur when you find your thoughts drifting to loved ones and you begin to worry about their future, or you notice a pain in your abdomen and your mind jumps to the worst-case scenario. There are things that cause stress and make most of us anxious, such as family situations, finances, personal health, social events and conflict, but so many things are our own personal triggers.

You may find journaling to be a helpful tool in discerning where and when stress and anxiety are triggered for you. Even the act of journaling has been found to reduce these unpleasant states. When we write and reflect, it quiets the amygdala and engages the pre-frontal cortex, which means that our access to problem solving and creative thinking open up.

Mindful Tip: *Another benefit of journaling is that sometimes we have the opportunity to reflect and realize that we're not always rational, and that both stress and anxiety come and go like waves on the ocean. When we can remind ourselves of this during times of anxiousness, it may help to reduce some of the energetic charge around our feelings and experience. Hence the wise saying, "This too, shall pass."*

If it is supportive for you and feels right, you may want to list some of the things that would help to reduce your stress. Here is a sample of what that might look like:

Headaches: Make appointment with doctor

- Note to self: STOP going on to WebMD as it only exacerbates my anxiety

Finances: Make appointment at financial institution or speak with my brother Rod who is responsible with money

Upcoming presentation: Ask Kerri at work to help me practice

Commuting: Listen to soothing music on the way in

World events: Give myself a time-out from media for a while

Cold medicine: Switch brands because this one makes me jittery and is giving me nightmares

Dinner at in-laws: Set better boundaries around how often we will visit

Triggers: Call my organization's Employee and Family Assistance Program or make an appointment with the therapist that Laurie suggested

Other notes: Eat regularly, as I noticed that I get jittery and on-edge when I skip meals, check out self-compassion videos on YouTube to help me be kinder with myself, picture a STOP sign when I notice that I'm worrying about work again, and then focus my thoughts on how great my garden is doing and how much I love my dog, Lucy

If journaling is helpful for you, that's great to know. If journaling is not helpful for you, that's great to know, too. Find the tools and resources that feel like a good fit, and don't force anything that doesn't feel right.

Free Resources: *According to www.healthline.com, the following apps are said to be the best for dealing with anxiety, all of which are free to download, but may have a monthly fee in order to access some of all of the content:*

- **Best anxiety app for meditation:** Calm
- **Best anxiety app for adult coloring:** Colorfy
- **Best for mood tracking:** What's Up? A Mental Health App
- **Best anxiety app for sleep:** Nature Sounds Relax and Sleep
- **Best meditation app for People of Color:** Shine
- **Best anxiety app for breathing techniques:** Breathwrk
- **Best anxiety app game:** AntiStress Anxiety Relief Game
- **Best anxiety app for journaling:** Moodnotes
- **Best for cognitive behavioral therapy (CBT):** MindShift CBT

"The most difficult thing is the decision to act. The rest is merely tenacity."

– Amelia Earhart

Part V: The Why

"I like living. I have sometimes been wildly, despairingly, acutely miserable, wracked with sorrow, but through it all I still know quite certainly that just to be alive is a grand thing."

– Agatha Christie

Suffering from stress or anxiety can sometimes leave a person wondering if there is something wrong with them. I have found that for many people, understanding where these states come from – *why* we feel the way we do, and the fact that there are scientific reasons for it – has played an enormous role in releasing the strangle hold that feeling out of control can have on a person. It can truly be liberating to finally understand *why* we do the things we do, so that the internal blame-game of "what's wrong with me?" can finally shift to, "Oh, I see what's happening here; what can I do in order to best support myself in this moment of suffering?"

Stress and anxiety actually have deep evolutionary and biological roots that make perfect sense, so let's investigate just a few of them and see if we can loosen and reduce some anxiety around feeling at times like we might be "going crazy."

Firstly, it is imperative that we understand that humans did not evolve to be happy; humans evolved to survive. From a biological perspective, that was our entire purpose.

Evolution: Example #1

This journey into evolution takes us back a few million years ago to our more primitive lizard days. There wasn't a lot that a lizard needed to know much more than "Do I eat it, or does it eat me?" (Aside from, "Can I mate with it?") The brain of this lizard was wired to either fight (if it was something that the lizard would eat or compete with), flee (if it was something that was going to eat the lizard), freeze (if options were limited and it needed to hide or play dead in order to save itself from being eaten), or faint (if death was likely or imminent). Hence, the fight/flight/freeze/faint response that we hear about, more often just shortened to fight, flight and freeze or to flight or fight.

As we evolved over time, humans grew the capacity to think – we began to remember things that were important and to strategize in order to ensure that we would be able to have enough food not just for the present day, but also for the days and seasons to come. This adaptation was vital to the survival of our species.

There were two significant types of errors that our ancestors could make back then. The first type of error was thinking that something could hurt them when actually it couldn't. For example, this ancestor could see something out of the corner of their eye, such as a rock, and mistake it for a tiger. It would give them a scare, but wouldn't amount to much. The second type of error was thinking that something couldn't hurt them when it could. For example, they could see something out of the corner of their eye, such as a tiger, and mistake it for a rock. This type of error would cost the human their life. The humans that didn't think that things were going to hurt them did not survive; they are not our ancestors. Our lineage, the lineage of all human beings, comes from the ancestors that were constantly on the lookout for stuff that could hurt them. The human brain grew around concepts such as looking out for the berries that would poison them, the members of other tribes that would compete with them for food or mates, and the predators that would jump out and eat them. Hence, humans evolved to be on the lookout for the "bad." This phenomenon has been named by scientists to be our "Negativity Bias." No, I am not joking. If this is not something you have heard of before, it's a real thing. Humans are programmed to look for the negative: This was supportive of our survival as a species, but not supportive for our levels of happiness.

Quick Tip: *If you are someone that experiences stress or anxiety because you tend to focus on the negative side of things, rest assured that this is a normal biological adaptation that all humans possess; you are normal. Luckily, the Negativity Bias that we all have can be reprogrammed*

Mindful Exercise: One Good Thing

The world has changed faster than the human brain could adapt, meaning that we no longer have to be on the lookout to the same degree for plants that will poison us, tribes that will compete with us and predators that will eat us, but the recesses of our brains don't necessarily know this yet. The wonderful news is that we can take simple, easy steps to rewire our brains to be less anxious and to release our hold on the need to be on the lookout for the negative. Just as humans changed our biology in order to look for the negative, we can also adapt our brains to look for the positive. We can literally train our brains to overcome our hardwired Negativity Bias.

1) If it feels comfortable for you, allow your eyes to close, or to softly gaze at something without focusing on it too much

2) Bring to your mind's eye to one thing that is good in your life. It could be anything, such as a person or pet that you care for, a good memory, a prized

possession, something in nature that you enjoy, a vacation spot that brings you pleasure, something that you like about yourself. Perhaps it is that you love to eat peanut butter and jam on toast. It can be anything at all that is "good" – big or small. Bring to mind One Good Thing

3) Stay with this One Good Thing. Linger in it for at least 20 to 30 seconds, really getting a feel for how much you enjoy it. Allow this sensation or feeling(s) to sink into you, as though you are a sponge that is soaking up these good feelings

4) If you notice that more than one good thing is coming to mind, allow that thing or those things to come into your awareness as well. Really savor the sensations and emotions that arise

5) When you are ready, create an intention to look for, and notice more good things in your daily life

6) When you have completed this practice, consider smiling and stretching as you open your eyes or return to your normal gaze

That's it! That's how simple it can be for us to begin to access the plasticity of our brains. We can literally rewire our brains for less negativity and more positivity. These things are cumulative – they add up. The more the better. Consider looking, and even searching for everyday things that are "good" in life. This could be a green light when you are in a hurry to drive somewhere, a sunset, the smell of freshly cut grass, the sound of a loved one laughing, or indulging in the sense of relief when you sit down on the couch at the end of a busy day. Remember to really soak in the good before moving on. If we look for them, there are One Good Thing's all around us.

> **Free Resource:** *Dr. Rick Hanson has a free e-newsletter that gets published on a regular basis with unlimited suggestions for overcoming the Negativity Bias, as well as lots of other useful information for living a happier, healthier life. At the time of publishing, he also runs weekly on-line meditations on Wednesdays. Find out more or sign up for the e-newsletter or meditations at www.rickhanson.net.*

But Does it Work?

Years ago, when my kids were out playing basketball, Liz threw the ball at the basket and then reached down to tie her shoe. Unbeknownst to both of them, there was a wasp nest just behind the backboard. The wasps came out with a fury, and with Liz bent down in front of him, they went straight for my son, Jonathon. He was stung several times, including multiple stings to the face.

As the days and weeks moved on, Jonathon (understandably) became increasingly agitated by the sight of wasps, to the point that if we were out on the deck having dinner and one flew past, he would quickly go inside and refuse to eat with us. The avoidance of wasps then shifted to *all* bugs, and the anxiety inflated to a point where even the sight of a bug would send him into the dysregulated state of flight (and he would run away from wherever we were). Seeing that the issue was getting much worse versus better over time, something had to be done. I explained to him that this is one of the many ways that mental illness can take hold of us; the mind is trying to protect the body, but goes into overdrive in its goal to do so. His mind needed some support and resources, and it needed an intervention. Jonathon agreed that he would consciously and purposely search for bugs, and take note of when they were *not* trying to hurt him. His job was to notice them flying, or resting on a flower, or swarming around a public garbage can and to allow it to sink and soak in when the bugs were *not* there to harm him.

A few weeks after his new assignment, Jonathon came in from the yard, "Mom – I just saw the coolest thing! A wasp stung a spider and was dragging it across the dirt; spider still moving and everything! I got down close to get a better look and could see the huge spider getting more and more paralyzed. I've never seen anything like it!" He had completely forgotten that he was ever afraid of wasps.

> **<u>Mindful Tip:</u>** *Even if you have mental illness in the family, indicating that it may be in your genetic makeup, according to Genetic Researcher Kara Fitzgerald, genes are not our destiny; what <u>regulates</u> our genes (epigenetics) is our destiny. That means*

that our everyday choices, such as diet, sleep routines, interpersonal relationships, internal and environmental toxins, and stress loads all play a significant part in both our health-span (the amount of time in our lives that we benefit from good mental and physical health) and our life-span. Taking simple steps to reduce stress and anxiety can be the difference between which genes are activated and which genes are not. In fact, research supports the finding that even one meditation practice or self-regulating activity can favorably change gene expression

Evolution: Example #2

Humans evolved to avoid pain. This makes complete sense from a biological standpoint, as pain often equated to getting hurt, and getting hurt could often equate to dying. Hence, if our ancestors were able to avoid pain, they lived. Not only did humans use memory in order to avoid danger and pain, they also used strategy. This is where the rubber really hits the road for anxiety; if our ancestors could strategize well enough, using their Negativity Bias, continuation of the lineage was more likely. If your anxiety shows up in ways that have you ruminating over all of the bad things that *could possibly* happen in the future, you are not alone, and you come by it honestly – through evolution. I've found that rumination is one of the most common complaints when it comes to people feeling as though their mental health is declining. What starts as often a responsible person just "planning" for what could go wrong can quickly escalate and get out of hand, with worrisome thoughts taking over much of their time and energy, robbing them of joy.

As difficult as it can seem, a large part of breaking the cycle of rumination is to stop ruminating. This can sound like an impossible task to those of us who have been "planning" scenarios in order to feel safer, and there may even be some hesitancy in wanting to stop, because there can be a sense of familiarity and even safety in feeling so unsafe all of the time (we like that we are so antsy because it keeps us "on our toes"). Remember that we humans have brain plasticity – we can change the shape of our brains through new thoughts, feelings and experiences. This is true for those of us who ruminate as well.

Mindful Exercise: The STOP Practice

Breaking free from the tyranny of rumination takes some time and practice, just as it took time and practice to get so good at ruminating in the first place. Mindfulness is an integral part of breaking the cycle.

The first thing to do when you notice that you are caught in a thought process of negativity (whether about the future or the past) is to become aware of the fact that you are noticing it, "Oh, look at me! I'm caught in ruminative thinking again!" (No judgement, just kindly taking note of the fact that you are caught in a cycle of thinking that is not helpful for you.) Then STOP.

Stop what you are thinking about

Take a few breaths. Really allow yourself to sense the breath in your body – what does the air feel like as it enters through your nose, and as your body expands on the inhale? Become immersed in the sensation of your breath as you allow your body to relax

Observe what is happening for you in the moment without judgement. Without getting caught up in a storyline, what type of thoughts are you having? ("Hmmm…worrying about work again.") Observe the situation that led you to this thought process, or perhaps observe the physical sensations, such as tightness in the body, that are present for you

Proceed thoughtfully. What would be the best course of action from here? Is there something else that you can direct your attention to? Is there something else that you could do that would be more beneficial for yourself or others? Can you choose to purposely select a different thought pattern?

The goal here is to 1) Become mindful of the fact that you are caught up in a negative action or thought pattern 2) Interrupt the negative thought pattern by placing your awareness and focus on your breath 3) Connecting with how you feel so that you become more familiar with the sensations of being swept away in these patterns 4) Choosing to find a different focus for your awareness.

Free Resource: *Dr. Joe Dispenza is the best-selling author of "Breaking the Habit of Being Yourself" and "You are the Placebo" and has lots of interesting and inspirational material on YouTube regarding brain plasticity and creating new thought patterns and habits*

On a personal note, I use the STOP Practice on a regular basis. One such way is whenever I find myself worrying about flooding in our home, as we had several issues when the house was being built (and The Negativity Bias rears its ugly head every so often), leading me to have anxious thoughts that it may happen again. As soon as I catch myself in this stressful thought pattern, I STOP. I take a few deep breaths, and observe that my mind has been carried away again and that my chest is tight. Then I purposely choose (proceed thoughtfully) to think about something else – whether it is simply a more pleasant thought pattern, or something that I could be doing that is a better use of my time. It wasn't always easy at first, but has become much easier and faster with practice.

Quick Tip: *Where attention goes, energy flows. The more attention that we give to negative thought patterns, they larger they seem to get, often flooding our awareness and hijacking our energetic resources. When we purposely select different and more helpful thought patterns, our energy follows that attention, freeing up our* *resources for thoughts and feelings that are more supportive for overall health and well-being. (It is not about denying how you feel, it is simply about consciously choosing thoughts that are more nourishing for you.)*

I also use the STOP Practice quite regularly with one of my adolescent children. My daughter has an issue with being on time – in that it is difficult for her (although, admittedly, she is getting much better). When I find myself losing my cool because we are late (again) due to waiting for her (again), as soon as I notice my temper flaring, I say to myself, STOP, STOP, STOP! This serves two purposes – the first is to stop me in my tracks if I am about to raise my voice (or am in the middle of raising my voice) and the second is as a reminder for me to take a breath and proceed with a better choice than getting angry or impatient, and possibly saying something that I would later regret. In this way, I have used the STOP Practice as a form of neuro-linguistic programming, in that the moment I think the word STOP I immediately (literally mid-sentence at times) cease what I am doing. This now happens automatically from regular practice of the technique.

Evolution: Example #3

"The goal is not to be better than the other man, but your previous self"

The Dalai Lama

Another form of stress that can be quite overwhelming (in addition to The Negativity Bias and ruminative thinking) is over-identification around the concern of what other people are thinking about us. You are not alone if the worry of how others view you causes you great strife in your life. Yet again, we can thank our ancestors for this. Evolutionarily speaking, the dominant animals and humans were the ones that were more likely to survive and procreate. The more dominant, the more access they would have to resources and mates, and the more protection that would be available for their offspring. Our genes have been programmed with the desire to be the winner…of everything. This can create a relentless concern with self-esteem. This form of anxiety equates to possibly being over-concerned with things like money, looks, brains, strength, perceived power and position (including fame) and all other ego-related things. ("What do they think of me? Do they think I'm attractive? How do they view my work? How many 'likes' did I get today?" – the endless list can be another source of constant rumination.) Even wanting to be regarded as "the nicest" or kindest person, or the most spiritually evolved can serve to feed a person's desire for ego fulfilment. It also means that when people *do* say or act in ways that can be construed as a threat to ego, that a person can literally experience feelings of being "under attack" (which could trigger the fight, flight or freeze response).

Finding Your Own Perfect Fit:

Many years ago, while attending a week-long meditation retreat at a well-known Centre, I had trouble utilizing the main meditation technique taught by the 'guru'. Others went around talking about how wonderful the technique worked, and shared stories of deep, meaningful and touching meditations, but try as I might, I just couldn't get there: *What is wrong with me? How come everyone else can get this and I can't? Am I stupid or something?* I was just as hung up (if not more so) about myself in comparison to the others in the group as I was on the fact that what I was doing wasn't working.

Finally, I couldn't take it anymore and switched to a different meditation technique that seemed more authentic for me. Sure enough, my body relaxed and I was able to reach a much deeper level of meditation. Every so often throughout the years I've gone back to give that old technique a try in order to see if now I finally "get it," but to no avail: Even if a technique seems to work for *everyone* except you, I invite you to honor that it doesn't work for you. As soon as I stopped caring about the fact that I was different and wasn't "getting it" (stopped caring about myself in comparison to others), I was able to settle into the techniques and practices that were right for me. If you haven't found your right fit yet, it does not mean that there is anything wrong with you; it is simply an invitation to keep looking – your perfect fit it out there, even if it's different from what works for others. Besides, we don't improve our physical fitness by doing the same thing every day; we need new exercises, new reps and new intensities in order to continue our growth and development. Being able to match self-care interventions to how we are feeling is a skill that is acquired through trial and error, and doesn't ever need to be done in comparison with what works for others.

> **Mindful Tip:** *Comparing oneself to others is such an unnecessary and painful, anxiety-provoking choice. Remember that it is a choice, and that you do not have to make comparisons. Also remember that others often make a big production of publicly sharing their highlight reels, but are much less open with their blooper reels. 'Staying in your own lane' is a recipe for less anxiety or stress and greater health and wellbeing*

If this form of anxiety rings true for you, that's okay, and good for you for recognizing that. Fortunately, we have other mental capacities that can counteract this preoccupation with ego as well. The pivotal part to changing, though, is changing – and that includes what we do and how we think.

Mindful Practice: Inquiry of the Ego

Egos are an important and integral part of being human. It is with the help of our ego that we decide what we will put up with and what we won't – our ego helps us to define what matters to us, and to create healthy boundaries. That being said, it is important and helpful to become familiar with one's ego; to befriend it in order to create a more intimate relationship with oneself. The following exercise may be helpful in seeing the different faces of ego – realizing the difference between how others view you and how you view yourself, as well as what matters most to you.

I Am

- Find a comfortable place to sit where you won't be disturbed and allow your eyes to close or softy gaze

- Gently and quietly say or think to yourself, "I am (first name, last name)." For example, Tom Smith would think to himself, "I am Tom Smith."

- Without trying to force anything, see what arises for you in your awareness as you think this. What automatically comes to mind?

- When you are ready to move on, gently think or say to yourself, "I am (first name)." Tom Smith would now think, "I am Tom."

- Again, without "trying", just gently allow anything to float into your awareness. What comes up when you are no longer your first and last name?

- When you are ready, softly think or say to yourself, "I am." What arises for you when you are no longer your name? It is possible that you may not need words, descriptions, titles or pictures – it may be that you settle your awareness simply on a feeling, sensation or emotion.

- When you have finished investigating how that feels, kindly think or say to yourself, "I." That is all there is. You don't need to be anything else. How do you feel and what comes up for you?

- Lastly, when you are ready, investigate what it feels like to let go of the "I". What is it like for you to "be" without having to be anyone?

- Gently allow your eyes to slowly open if they were closed and take some time before moving again into "doing."

If at any time during that exercise you feel uncomfortable, then as always, know that you have complete agency and choice; you can change the practice or stop it. These mindful exercises are all simply invitations for you to try something that may or may not work for you, and to go from there. I believe that meditation can be like a buffet – give things a little try and see what you're in the mood for in that moment.

> **Mindful Reminder:** *You are not your emotions. You are not your beliefs. You are not the story you tell yourself. You are the magnificent energetic being that is aware of your emotions, your beliefs and your stories*

Biology: Example #4

In truly grasping an understanding of anxiety, it is also important to know a little about our biology.

When we become triggered with the nervous system activation of a "fight or flight" response, there are numerous reactions that occur within the body, and the majority of them all take place within less that a second's time.

Let's go back to our friend Tom Smith for this. If Tom wakes up in the middle of the night to a loud crash, and assumes that there is a burglar in his home, his body will unconsciously and automatically prepare him for the fight or flight that is about to take place:

- Pupils dilate in order to increase peripheral vision, because history predicts that predators tend to attack from the side more often than the front
- Hearing immediately shifts so that lower frequency noises (such as footsteps on the stairs) can be more

readily heard (making it more difficult to hear "regular voices or talking")

- Mouth becomes dry, as inner resources are shifted from the priority of "rest and digest" to "fight or flight" – having access to saliva in order to break down food takes a back seat as those internal resources are mobilized for more pressing matters
- Jaw tenses as Tom bears down to run or fight
- Changes in the throat make for a male's voice to be louder and deeper in order intimidate his attacker. As a throw-back to the old days, a female's voice will become higher and shriller in order for her to yell for help
- In another automatic attempt to look fiercer to an adversary, the shoulders move up closer to the ears so that Tom comes off as more menacing
- Fists clench in order to make punching or running more efficient
- The heart begins to beat faster in an effort to move blood more readily throughout the body – muscles receive more oxygen so that they are stronger for fighting or running with
- Breathing becomes quick and shallow, again in an effort to increase oxygen intake
- Muscles tense in an effort to prepare the individual to sprint or enter into combat
- Sensing in hands and feet is reduced so that Tom is not slowed down from the pain of striking or

attacking another or the pain of being cut during a flee
- Feet shrink so that if engaged in battle, it is easier for one to maneuver
- Internally, the blood thickens so that if Tom is cut during battle or fleeing, his wounds clot faster and more efficiently

These are just a few of the many ways that the body automatically responds to stress. These unconscious changes to one's biology often would have meant the difference between life and death to our ancestors. Indeed, if there was an intruder in the house, these energetic injections are necessary.

However, let's say that Tom soon discovers that the loud crash was simply that his cat came running through the cat door, and that everything is fine. Normally, the body would work to return to homeostasis (the health of "home base" when all is calm in the body), which may include some shaking (in order to expel the mobilized energy that didn't end up getting used) or in tears (both of which are normal, unconscious and automatic mammalian responses to calm the body down and release excess energy) that should not be thwarted if at all possible.

What does all of this have to do with just regular, run-of-the-mill stress or anxiety? Well, Tom could quite easily trigger his fight or flight reflexes simply by receiving a nasty email, an unexpected bill in the mail, a passing glimpse from a co-worker that seems less than friendly, or a disagreement with his spouse. He could also trigger this response with his *thoughts.* As the brain cannot tell the difference between what is actually happening and what is thought to be happening, it will respond as though it is under attack. This response could be triggered by worrying about a loved one, thinking about all of the items on a to-do list or rehashing a conversation that he wished had gone differently. The brain senses a threat and the body becomes mobilized for action. That means that these regular run-of-the-mill everyday occurrences can shift the body into the same reactionary state as if we had to flee from or fight off an intruder. If the mind is stressful, the body will follow. The same is true if that if the body is stressful, the mind will follow. As Polyvagal Theory expert Deb Dana says, "Physical state creates a psychological story." That means that when the body is stressed and anxious, the mind becomes stressed and anxious, and will create stressful and anxious thoughts. The sticky part here is that as the mind creates stressful and anxious thoughts, the body becomes more stressed and anxious – the cycle perpetuates itself until the energy can be dispelled, which, for some people, may not take place until after a full-blown panic attack or rage-event has occurred.

Thankfully, there is much that can be done to counteract all of this. The first step is to become educated (as you are now) and the second step is to use mindfulness to recognize what is happening as it happens. Previously, we have discussed ways of interrupting negative thought patterns in order to quiet upsetting thoughts, and now we want to look at the other piece of the puzzle – calming the body so that it doesn't unwittingly trigger anxious (or stressful, or depressive, etc.) thoughts.

Mindful Practice: Conscious Relaxation

When we consciously relax the body, it sends communication to the brain that we are safe. In effect, purposely relaxing overrides the bodily system to let it know that the fight or flight response is not necessary. (As with the other Mindful Practices, you may wish to use the voice memo option on your phone to record yourself slowly and quietly reading out these instructions - with a long pause between each one - so that you are not having to go back and forth between reading and practicing.)

- Find a comfortable place to sit where you will not be disturbed. (If sitting is not physically supportive, feel free to lie down, although staying awake can sometimes be a challenge with this exercise.) Close your eyes if that feels comfortable, or lower them to a soft gaze

- Allow your breathing to gently find itself as you let go of the day and bring your focus to yourself and your body

- Connect with the top of your head and see if you can sense any tingling or other sensations on your head. Now imagine the top of your head relaxing

- Allow your forehead to let go

- Bring your awareness to your eyes. Become aware of whether or not they feel strained. Invite your eyes, to relax and let go. Imagine that even the back of your eyeballs let go of any tension

- Consciously release any tension from your eyebrows or the middle of your eyes

- Invite your earlobes to relax

- Release your jaw

- Relax your neck

- Allow your shoulders to melt away from your neck. Sense the feeling of gravity gently pulling at the heaviness of your arms in order for you to release even further

- Soften your arms from your shoulders to your hands

- Invite your fingers to relax, including the finger tips

- Become aware of your chest. Breathe slowly and deeply as you relax your chest

- If you notice any thoughts or resistance arising at any time, simply say to yourself gently, "Nowhere to be. Nothing to do." Then bring your awareness back to your body and continue to relax (This may take several reminders, just be gentle and loving with yourself)

- Sense your belly. Soften the belly. Relax your intestines and visceral organs. Breath slowly, deeply and softly into your belly if it is comfortable for you. It may feel fitting for you to gently say to yourself, "Nobody to impress – nothing to hold in."

- Relax the back. Feel your back slowly expand and contract with your breath. It may feel nourishing to gently think to yourself, "I do not have to carry the weight of the world right now. I am releasing."

- Consciously relax your hips

- Release the muscles in the buttocks and glutes

- Allow your legs to feel heavy and supported as you purposely unstiffen the muscles

- Relax the feet, including the toes and tips of the toes

- Become aware of your entire body. Release anything that has unconsciously stiffened again. Imagine that even your skin is relaxing

- Savor this sensation of being entirely relaxed. Imagine that this ease is rewriting your DNA

- Softly say or think to yourself, "This is what it feels like to be relaxed"

- When you are ready, open your eyes or raise your gaze slowly, curiously investigating if you are still able to keep a sense of quiet, stillness, calmness or relaxation as you begin to engage in your outer world again

That was the long version. A shorter version is simply:

Mindful Exercise: Conscious Relaxation – Short Version

- Sitting or standing comfortably, allow your face to soften, including eyes, cheeks, and jaw. Feel your tongue gently resting at the roof of your mouth behind the teeth

- Release your shoulders as you feel gravity helping to move them away from your neck

- Relax your torso as you breath slowly and deeply – this includes the chest, back and belly

- Soften the muscles from your hips to the bottom of your feet

Often, when we sense stress or anxiety swelling, we tense our bodies, which only serves to make things worse: the mind controls the body and the body controls the mind. As soon as we gain control of one, we can control the other. As with all of the exercises in this guide, the more you practice this, the easier it becomes. In fact, it is possible for your body to relearn that instead of being stressed or anxious, the new homeostasis is to be relaxed. The benefits of this default are too numerous to count, not the least of which is that a relaxed body promotes a relaxed mind which greatly and significantly reduces levels of stress and anxiety.

Mindful Tip: *When you experience stress or anxiety, curiously investigate if there is any part of you that is not stressed or anxious in that moment. Even if it is your hair, or your belly button, or your pinky toe, try putting your attention there and then gently exploring if it is at all possible for that feeling to expand outward*

There are many times when the body will have a reaction that may stimulate feelings of stress or anxiety unnecessarily. Below is a very short list of some of the daily occurrences that can make your body "think" that you are stressed, when it is not true:

- Waking up. Not kidding. The body automatically provides a boost of cortisol upon waking in order to mobilize us for the day. This is especially noticeable for highly sensitive people. You may wake up with your heart beating quickly and your chest tightened and assume that you are just "naturally anxious." This is easily overcome by taking a moment to breathe slowly and deeply in bed for a moment as you say to yourself, "Oh, thank you for making sure that I am ready to start the day." (Always remember – just because you *feel* like you are stressed or anxious doesn't necessarily mean that you actually are! – Ask yourself, "Am I actually anxious right now, or is my body maybe just responding to something in the environment?") People may also experience this jolt of cortisol upon waking by swinging out to strike someone (some wake up feeling like they need to flee, others wake up feeling like they need to fight – that fact can easily affect mood if one is not paying attention)
- Consumption of caffeine. Depending on how sensitive you are, caffeine can trigger a full nervous system activation, including sweating from the palms, forehead or underarms, heart pounding and quickened breathing. If you are not mindful of the fact that you are having a reaction to caffeine, your brain may trigger anxious thoughts in your mind,

such as, "How am I ever going to get all of this work done?" or "I made such a fool out of myself the other day! What will they think of me?" (Personal default has a lot to do with the flavor of one's stressful thoughts)

- Consumption of too many carbs or too much sugar (including the sugar in fruit). This will get the heart pounding as the body works to take care of the ingested toxin, which can feel very similar to anxiety
- Any form of bodily tension (which is why we just practiced conscious relaxation). Even if the body is tense because of a kink in the neck, it may trigger anxious thoughts (in order to get your mind to match your body). Again, simply asking yourself, "Am I actually anxious right now, or is my body just trying to tell me something?" can be very helpful
- Skipping meals. When we get hungry, our amygdala can sense a threat due to lack of food (hence people who get "hangry" because their fight has been activated). Also, if you tend to get the shakes when you're hungry, that could activate anxious thinking
- Daily/monthly hormonal fluctuations. This is not specifically just for females, nor is it specifically around menstruating, PMS, ovulation, peri-menopause or menopause. Regular, monthly hormonal fluctuations happen in any body, in any gender at any given time. If one is not mindful of this, it may trigger thoughts of anxiety, paranoia, sadness, anger, etc.

- Further to the point listed above, anything that affects hormones (stress, vitamins, missing meals, low testosterone, adrenal fatigue, improper diet including not enough protein, lack of sleep, illness, etc.) can cause one to feel as though they have been triggered into stress or anxiety
- Certain prescription drugs or OTC prescriptions including birth control pills, cough/cold medications and weight-loss pills
- Consumption of any toxins including alcohol, nicotine, drugs, etc.

You get the point. Almost anything that we do can trigger a fight or flight (sympathetic nervous system) activation. That's okay – our bodies are designed to be able to be triggered and then to move back into homeostasis. We can just help our bodies along by recognizing when we have been bounced out of "rest and digest" (parasympathetic nervous system) and then taking whatever step or steps work best for us in order to bring us back into our resting state, which can be a simple as merely eliciting a yawn.

Mindful Tip: *Yawning has tremendous health benefits, including the fact that it interrupts the brain's release of stress-stimulating neurochemicals and immediately helps one to feel calmer. Yawn before an exam. Yawn if you are having anxious thoughts. Yawn if you are feeling stress over tasks that need to be completed. Can't yawn on cue? Watch someone else yawn (even on*

YouTube) or fake a few in a row and an authentic yawn is likely to follow

When we are feeling stressed, it is an amazing communication from either the body or the mind that something in our system has become dysregulated. As we've just investigated, it could be that the dysregulation has occurred innocently because of something that we have consumed, or thought, or a change in our hormones, but it could be due to other things as well. The point is that stress and anxiety are like the check engine light of the brain – if the light didn't go off, we wouldn't know that there was a problem… until it was too late. In fact, stress and anxiety are not our enemy – they are our protectors, simply communicating that something needs to be addressed in order to support a higher level of health and wellbeing.

Mindful Tip: *Instead of viewing anxiety as your enemy, consider viewing it as your faithful helper and lovingly say to it, "Thank you for being here! What is it that you're trying to tell me?" You may find that your faithful helper has a real point – something that truly is a threat that needs to be addressed - or perhaps your helper has been a little too keen in sensing a problem and you can let it know that everything is okay*

We do not want to ignore stress or deny that we are feeling anxious – doing that is like covering the check engine light in your car and then acting like the situation has been resolved. An integral part of overcoming anxiety is to validate its existence in the first place. It has a purpose: What is your stress or anxiety wanting to communicate to you? Wherever your anxiety is coming from and no matter what message it is trying to convey to you, it makes sense. Maybe your stress or anxiety are trying to ensure that you don't embarrass yourself in front of others, or that you don't fail at something. Maybe they don't want you to look stupid or to get into trouble. Maybe the message is that two cups of coffee is your limit. Maybe the message is that you need to nourish your body more often with relaxation. Perhaps it's that you need more sleep, less work, better food, more exercise, or thoughts that are affirming versus negating and self-deprecating. It is possible that your stress is trying to communicate to you that it is time to set better boundaries, to exit a relationship that isn't nourishing for you, or to enlist the help of a professional because there are things that you are dealing with (or not dealing with) that you need support with. Your job is simply to figure out why the "check engine" light is on, and you might need to enlist the support of a mechanic (subject matter expert) to help you in getting to the root of the issue.

Mindful Tip: *Saying to yourself or to anyone struggling with stress or anxiety the simple statement, "That makes sense" is an excellent tool for calming the nervous system and regulating brain* *function so that rational thought can prevail. Then, the mystery of what the stress is wanting to communicate can be solved more effectively*

Biology: Example #5

Let's continue investigating human biology as we take an even deeper dive into the inner workings of the nervous system.

Imagine that your nervous system is like a teeter-totter. When the teeter-totter of your nervous system is up (sympathetic arousal) then you may feel anxious, irritable, edgy, or restless. Basically, it can feel like you just want or need to "go-go-go!". When the teeter-totter of your nervous system is down (dorsal parasympathetic arousal) then you may feel sluggish, numb, uninterested, immobilized or depressed. Basically, it can feel like you just don't want or need to move. When the seesaw is in the middle (ventral parasympathetic nervous system) then you are feeling pretty balanced; like for the most part you can handle life and whatever it throws at you.

When you're feeling stressed, this indicates that your seesaw is not balanced. The first thing to do here is to ask yourself, "Am I up right now, or am I down?" because the interventions for each of the activations can, at times, be quite different.

If you find that you are feeling like your teeter-totter is down, you may find yourself procrastinating, and often when we procrastinate there can be another layer to add to an already existent feeling of weight: shame. There are times when procrastination is simply procrastination – we honestly just don't want to do something. But there are other times when procrastination is a fear response, except stuck on the "down" (not wanting to do anything) instead of being stuck on the "up" (wanting to do everything). The importance of knowing these things and differentiating between what really is happening inside of you and what you *think* is happening inside of you is that not knowing what's going on can leave a person thinking that they are lazy or unmotivated, or that something else is inherently wrong with them.

Once we know *why* something is happening, it is time to turn to the *how* you are going to handle it. The solution begins again with self-kindness and compassionate self-talk.

Mindful Tip: *Self-compassion has been researched and proven to be an effective way to motivate oneself and to become better connected to oneself and others*

When we speak harshly to ourselves, our nervous system detects a threat and then throws our body into a deeper state of activation, further perpetuating the effects of anxiety and stress. Often, an effective way of dealing with anxiety is to simply speak to yourself in a kind and loving manner in order to support what your body needs from you.

Free Resource: *Take the self-compassion quiz and find loads of information regarding self-compassion at Dr. Kristin Neff's website: www.self-compassion.org*

Mindful Exercise: Movement and Resonance

If you notice that your nervous system has been dysregulated, trying using this visual exercise of resonance:

- Connect with how you are feeling internally

- Using hand motions as a representation (such as wringing, shaking, fists, etc.), show yourself how you are feeling on the inside

- When it feels comfortable for you to proceed, now use hand motions to represent how you would *like* to feel on the inside using a soothing rhythm while taking long, slow, deep breaths and allowing your body to relax (if it feels comfortable, consider using your body as well as your hands to portray the sense that you would like to embody

You may find that becoming physical through the use of your hands and then providing for yourself a physical representation of how you would like to feel that your physiology follows.

Mindful Reflection: *Releasing any pull to get caught up in pain or emotion from the past, factually reflect upon how you were treated while growing up and developing a sense of self. If you were treated without care, as though you were not worth anything, then it is likely that you have developed to treat yourself as though you are worthless. If you were brought up in a household that was harsh, or were treated harshly, then it is likely that you have developed to treat yourself harshly. We can rewrite the way that we treat ourselves by beginning the journey to treat ourselves differently; by treating ourselves with kindness, compassion, concern, respect, and love*

Biology: Example #6

Approximately 20 – 30% of the population falls under the category of being classified as highly sensitive. The term "Highly Sensitive Person" was popularized by Dr. Elaine Aron, American psychologist and author of many books including *The Highly Sensitive Person* and *The Highly Sensitive Child.* Highly

Sensitive People are biologically different from non-HSP's in many ways. Clearly, from an evolutionary point of view, these adaptations make sense, because if they didn't, the highly sensitive person would not be here today. High sensitivity is also found in nature; any herd benefits from the animals that will rush in to ensure that they are the first to the food, but also from the animals in the group that will be more hesitant in order to ensure that there are no predators waiting to strike. Non-Highly Sensitive People and animals and Highly Sensitive People and animals have evolved to support one another in ensuring the survival of the species. True to the name, Highly Sensitive People are highly sensitive. This means that they are already hard-wired to be more sensitive to sound, sight, smell, taste and touch. HSP's tend to have better peripheral vision in order to detect danger, faster startle responses in order to respond quicker to threat, and a larger pre-frontal cortex which supports their memory function in order to recall hazards. Most importantly for the purposes of this guide, Highly Sensitive People also have a larger amygdala. If you recall from chapter "The Where," the amygdala works as the brain's "smoke detector," constantly scanning for threats and then taking over if it detects danger. Hence, people who are highly sensitive are literally hard-wired to be more reactive to their environments, to be more sensitive to remembering the negative (a stronger Negativity Bias) and more alert and responsive to any real or perceived threat.

High Sensitivity is hereditary, so if there is someone in your family that is highly sensitive (mother, father, aunt, uncle, grandparent, etc.) there is a stronger likelihood that you could be highly sensitive, and hence, more prone to anxiety.

Familiarizing Yourself with Yourself: Are you a Highly Sensitive Person? (Place a check mark with all that apply)

- __ Have been told in your life that you have "thin skin"

- __ Are a light sleeper
- __ Have a very keen sense of smell, sometimes to the point of being nauseated by anything from perfume or cigarette smoke to household cleaners or body odor

- __ Are sensitive to light in ways such as finding things "too bright", "too dim", or not being able to calm down or concentrate if the lighting isn't "just right". You may find "wrong" lighting distracting, irritating, angering, or even saddening and depressing

- __ Have highly intense (roller-coaster) emotions around anything from being deeply hurt by everyday comments or "betrayals", to experiencing love, happiness or joy more than most people seem to

- __ Become overwhelmed physically by movement, especially after puberty. This may include amusement park rides, or carsickness and seasickness and possibly even things such as movies or programs with too much movement in them

- __ Have extreme sensitivity to temperature, such as overheating easily, becoming more cold or chilled than others, or having bodily responses such as a blotchy or beet red face from moderate exertion. Your fingernails might turn blue when you get cold

- __ Are driven crazy by things like creases in bedsheets, seams in socks, tags on clothing or having anything against your skin that "feels scratchy". You may have a severe dislike for wearing anything with even the smallest fraction of wool in it

- __ Bruise easily

- __ Take a longer time than others to heal for even small cuts or abrasions

- __ Are very sensitive to toxins such as caffeine, alcohol or normal prescription drugs and medicines (you may have been referred to as "cheap drunk" in your life)

- __ Can "feel" when the energy in a room is full of tension or lightness, or the atmosphere is about to change

- __ Have an acute sense of taste, in that you can pick out the slightest herb or spice or can tell when water, milk or other items "just taste different"

- __ Are the one in the household that gets asked to smell the food (meat, bread, soup, etc.) to see if it's "gone bad"

- __ Feel exhausted after being with others or in public, whether you're considered to be an introvert (more likely) or an extravert (less likely for HSP's, but still happens)

- __ Have an exaggerated startle response where you jump at noises that others don't, or people love to scare you because of your "overreaction"

- __ Prefer not to have to socialize with strangers and/or hate small talk

- __ Have difficulty masking your emotions, and may have been told that you have "a terrible poker face"

- __ Respond by speech either "too quickly" or "too slowly". We are either "too quick" because we are using our intuitive nature to finish the other person's sentence (in order to show them that we understand what they're trying to say, even though it's often not appreciated as it comes across as cutting them off), or "too slowly" because we are analyzing every single aspect of the situation before we respond in a "slow-motion/matrix" kind of way so that we are confident that our response will be accurate and thoughtful

- __ Are more bothered than others when you witness someone suffering or any type of injustice, whether it is in person, on television or in the newspaper

- __ Notice small or minute changes in your environment or in other people, such as the movement of a small item in someone's office, someone changing their normal earrings, someone you pass in the hall that has had a hair trimming, etc.

- __ Prefer to have one or two close friends in your inner circle versus lots of friends with whom you are not close

- __ Have difficulty controlling your tears. You tear up or cry in conversations or every-day life about things that do not seem to affect others at all

- __ Have a strong sense of intuition

- __ Are greatly bothered by movies, programs or stories that are scary, intense, suspenseful or violent

- __ Don't particularly like unnecessary change, such as being content eating the same breakfast/lunch every day and not liking to adjust habits/traditions

- __ Are a perfectionist

- __ Get overly anxious about things (you may recognize your Highly Sensitive Child on this one), such as "freak out" or have a panic attack when it is time for an immunization or blood test

- __ Dislike being the center of attention, especially in front of strangers. You don't enjoy public recognition at work and maybe deep down, don't even really like it when people sing the "Happy Birthday" song to you

- __ Prefer to wake up slowly and quietly, and find alarm clocks incredibly jarring and/or upsetting

- __ Can find some mouthwashes and toothpastes "too spicy"

- __ Are sensitive to sounds; this may include that you plug your ears when sirens go blasting by, are slightly agitated by public toilets that flush too loudly, or find certain people's voices to be like nails on a chalkboard

- __ May resort (or did in the past) to unhealthy coping mechanisms in order to "block out" excessive stimuli. This could include anything from excessive exercise or excessive nail biting and picking, to addictions with food, alcohol, drugs, spending, sex, work, etc. (Sometimes we HSP's will do anything to try to "be normal", "drown out the noise of life", or otherwise numb our senses)

If many of these things strike a chord with you (or someone you know), or even if a few of them are "very true" for you, then it is extremely likely that you are a Highly Sensitive Person. Although high sensitivity can cause you to be more prone to experience stress and anxiety, like all of the reasons for the root causes of anxiety, there are ways to befriend and overcome anxiousness. Personally, I am a highly sensitive person, as is my father and my two children – my father, my son and I have all found tools and techniques to overcome excessive anxiety (my daughter is still perfecting her toolkit).

Sometimes, simply knowing that you are highly sensitive, and thus more prone to anxiety can be just the validation that one needs in order to know that their overly stressed personality or anxiety is not in their head. That alone may offer some freedom from feeling like there is something inherently wrong with you. Stress is a real thing – again, the body's way of communicating that something needs to be addressed, even if simply acknowledged and comforted – and being highly sensitive is a gift. Like most gifts, there is a price tag, and that price tag is simply an invitation to support yourself and your highly sensitive needs. As with anyone who struggles with stress or anxiety, give yourself a break – you're only human.

> **Free Resource:** *Find out more about highly sensitive people at Elaine Aron's website: www.hsperson.com*

Biology: Example #7

Humans have sensory-motor brain cells called Mirror Neurons that are activated when we perform an action or witness another performing the same action. Hence, these cells "mirror" the actions of others. This is an adaptive evolutionary skill, as it provides us with a basis for compassion, and allows us to feel with another so that we can connect on a deeper, more emotional level. One of the most well-known examples of mirror neurons at play is yawning; when we witness another person (or possibly even another animal) yawning, we are often triggered to yawn as well. In fact, even reading the word 'yawn' can initiate the yawn response in people who are more sensitive. Another more graphic example would be those who gag or vomit by witnessing or even thinking about another person vomiting. Mirror neurons; part of being a primate.

Mirror neurons also come into play with the moods of others. You may be or know someone who cries when they witness the crying of another, or hear of another's misfortune. This means that we can in effect 'catch' the emotions of others. If we hear of someone who is anxious, are in physical proximity of someone who is anxious, or are emotionally connected to someone who suffers from stress, we ourselves can become anxious or stressed.

Scientific research has taught us that while some people, such as psychopaths and those with other personality disorders have less or no mirror neurons, others have been found to have these mirror neurons in excess. Specifically, people who score higher on the sensitivity spectrum are more likely to have a higher number of these neurons. Some individuals, most commonly referred to as 'Empaths' are known to have the highest levels of mirror neurons. In fact, these levels are so high that empaths not only sense the emotions of others, but actually *feel* these emotions as if they are their own. This can be an extremely confusing and overwhelming situation, especially if the empath is unaware of their abilities.

It is estimated that approximately 1% of the population are empaths, which would equate to roughly 80 million people globally. I, personally, believe this number to be painfully low, as many people are empaths without being aware that they are. Scientific studies have found that empaths are creative and resourceful people who are very good at coming up with adaptive and maladaptive ways of coping with their sensitivity, many of which are unconscious. Some empaths may cope by simply turning off their emotions (often at a young age) due to constant overwhelm, and others may turn to various addictions, especially using toxins such as drugs and alcohol in an effort to dull their senses, just to name two.

For example, as an empath myself, when I walk into a room of strangers, my chest will tighten and I will suddenly find it difficult to breathe if anyone in the room is anxious. Fortunately, I have often been very good at recognizing immediately who the emotion belongs to in order to center and calm myself. (However, as an empath, I also feel drawn to that person in an effort to offer comfort and to relieve their anxiety, but that is for another guide.) Even speaking to someone on the phone, sitting next to a stranger in a movie theatre, or passing someone in the mall can unexpectantly and immediately immerse an empath in a flood of emotions that are not actually their own. This is also true for physical empaths who sense not the emotions of others, but their physical symptoms, including those of a racing heart, tense muscles, and any other physical sensation that the person may be experiencing, as well as for telepathic empaths who can sense the stressful (and other) thoughts of others. Basically, empaths do not just feel *for* other people, more often than not, they feel *with* other people. In fact, scientific studies indicate that under certain circumstances empaths feel more discomfort than the person who is actually undergoing the painful or uncomfortable situation. This can leave empaths feeling anxious for a variety of reasons:

1) The empath feels and naturally embodies the stress or anxiety of the other person
2) The empath feels more anxiety for a situation than the other person feels themselves (fawning, etc.)

3) The empath is unaware that they are an empath and is stressed or anxious because they are suffering from what seem to be unpredictable mood swings, thoughts that do not make sense for them, or phantom pains that vanish as quickly as they arrive

If this resonates for you, or you feel that you know someone who may be empath, there is an abundance of information available on the internet in order for you to learn more about this sensitivity.

Mindful Tip: *Sometimes the best course of action is simply to remove yourself from the situation that you are in*

Mindful Practice: Is This Mine?

- Upon becoming aware of the fact that your mental, emotional or physical state has just dramatically changed without reason, center yourself. (This could be connecting with your breath, or the sensation of your feet on the ground, connecting with the image of an inanimate - and emotionless - object such as a rock or a stick, or any other grounding technique that works for you)

- When you feel more connected to yourself, slowly and silently ask, "Is this mine?" Often, the answer will float into your awareness. You may even sense an energy flow of who the emotion, thought, or sensation belongs to (for me, it feels like an invisible 'rope' that leads from my solar plexes directly to the person that I am sensing, whether they are in my presence or not)

- If the answer is not readily available, remain calm and grounded. Simply ask yourself, "Does this make sense for me in this moment?" Take a mental inventory of how you were feeling a moment ago, how you are feeling now, and what has just changed. (Were you just thinking about someone? Did you just enter a new location? Is there a person in your vicinity that was not there a moment ago?)

The more you practice this, the easier it will be. One of the best exercises for strengthening the ability to sense who different energies belong to is the same exercise that I recommend for building intuition: Mindful Body Awareness – connecting in with your body on a regular basis and non-judgmentally sensing where your muscles are tight and where they are soft. By memorizing how your body feels when it is calm and relaxed, you will become more tuned to detecting when your body is trying to communicate with you through tension and other sensations.

<u>Mindful Tip:</u> *Be diligent with regards to who you spend your time with, as consistently being in the presence of stressed or anxious people is incredibly likely to increase personal levels of stress and anxiety, especially for sensitive individuals that have high levels of mirror neurons*

History: Example #8

Regrettably, for far too many of us, to be human is to experience some type of trauma. Also regrettable, experiencing trauma can shift a person's propensity towards feeling stressed or anxious. Many people experience trauma that they are not even consciously aware of, such as trauma that occurred before speech was possible. One such type of trauma that thankfully is getting a lot of attention these days is the trauma that may have occurred earlier in life for people who were left to "cry it out" when they were babies. Forms of this include being "sleep trained" or "trained" to eat or void on a schedule. This type of neglect causes the baby to release stress hormones, which can quickly become a part of the person's wiring, affecting them for life until properly addressed. (For more information on the damaging effects of "training" babies, please check out the articles and information available on the topic at: www.psychologytoday.com) Of course, that's not the only form of trauma that can occur, and one of the many aftereffects of trauma is that it can hardwire a person to be susceptible to sensing threat, even when there is no threat present. It also hardwires the body to have a very low threshold of feeling safe in order to keep the person vigilant. This may present itself in a general sense of impending doom, or a belief that "the other shoe may drop at any time." If you find that this type of stress or anxiety rings true for you, rest assured that your flexible and adaptable biology along with your remarkable brain plasticity offer hope and freedom of what can feel like a life-sentence of fear.

> **Mindful Tip:** *If you know that there has been trauma in your family, that you have experienced trauma, or have had an adverse childhood experience (ACE), you can choose to be kinder to yourself in order to reduce your propensity towards stress, anxiety or illness*

Trauma is not something that should be dealt with on one's own. Finding a health professional that you resonate with is an integral part of healing. Choosing a specialist or specialists to work with is the same as choosing the tools for your "Overcoming Stress and Anxiety Toolkit" – you need to find what works for you. For example, to overcome post-traumatic stress disorder (PTSD) after a horrific car crash, I found great refuge with a psychologist who specialized in Self Regulation Therapy (SRT). A girlfriend of mine who had struggled with depression and anxiety for the majority of her life experienced relief with an expert in Cognitive Behavioural Therapy (CBT) and a member of my extended family that was struggling with anxiety and resentment around personal issues couldn't say enough about her gains of emotional freedom after working with a therapist who specialized in Dialectical Behavior Therapy (DBT). Another modality of therapy is Internal Family Systems (IFS), an opportunity to discover, explore, and befriend all of the different internal "parts" of us; the anxious parts and the brave parts, the protective parts and the permissive parts – the "parts" of us who make us who we are. Check out the cute, entertaining, and neurologically accurate animated movie "Inside Out" to get a humorous taste of what these different parts can look like. To learn more about IFS, check out Dr. Richard Schwartz's (author of *No Bad Parts*) website at www. https://ifs-institute.com. The options are unlimited, and help is out there. If you have access to an Employee and Family Assistance Program through work, I highly recommend that you give it a try. If financial difficulties are an issue, please look for the support that's available for you.

Free Resource: *It is common for males to feel less comfortable seeking mental health support than females. "Man Therapy" was designed to help reduce some of this stigma for men seeking support with mental health issues and uses humor in its interactive mental health campaign. If you are hesitant to reach out for help or looking to checkout a new, supportive tool, please take a look at: www.mantherapy.org*

Gratefully, we do not necessarily need to know the source of our trauma in order to heal from it. There are many modalities that can be used in order to train our bodies how to feel safe, and multiple options and techniques are still yet to be covered in this book, including healing properties that are already an innate part of our biology: Mammalian Comfort Techniques. As the name insinuates, these comfort techniques are common to all mammals and are intended to support our biology in returning to homeostasis. You may choose to give some of these exercises a test drive and see if anything resonates for you (think of a cat with her kittens and these techniques are likely to make sense immediately):

- **Soothing noises**. What does a cat do when you pat her or when she is nursing her kittens? She purrs. Why have we sung lullabies to babies throughout the ages? Because the soothing sounds are calming. When he's stressed, my husband loves to google and listen to things such as "Top ten singing auditions" for X Factor, American Idol, Britain's Got Talent, America's Got Talent, The Voice and more. Although he doesn't know it, this activity has been proven to calm the nervous system – simply listening to prosodic voices communicates to our internal operating system that we are safe. Some of the best soothing sounds we can receive are the ones we give to ourselves. One of the meditations that I teach that has received the most epic feedback is where I invite people to close their eyes and simply create a humming sound that feels comfortable for them. If anyone would like to accentuate the vibrations, I invite them to gently plug their ears. That's it. The class sits and creates long, low vibrational sounds for several minutes, yet people have described the experience as "life-changing." Many people have told me that the exercise provided them with the energetic release of tears. Once people get over the feeling of being embarrassed making sounds, it's a wonderful way to get to know their nervous system on a more intimate level. Lastly, many of us wish that someone or something could make our stress or anxiety better. *We* can make it better. Soothe yourself with the words that you need to hear right now. Either out loud or in your head, say or think those perfect sounds. "Everything will be okay." "You're safe, Sweetheart." "This too shall pass." "I have faith that good will come from this even though I can't see it right now." "You'll be alright, we'll make it through this together." Nobody knows the perfect things to murmur in order to comfort you better than you do. Even if it's an honest, "I don't know what to say right now, but I love you", that's perfect too.

- **Touch.** Pets and tame animals love to be patted. Horses, deer, lions all rub their faces together for comfort. Humans have skin sensors that are devoted only to sensing bodily warmth in another – humans are biologically designed to crave proximity and touch. The skin is our exposed nervous system and it is our job to calm our nervous system down. At time of publication, we are yet again facing another wave in the pandemic, but we can still hug and touch those that we feel comfortable with. Humans need touch no matter what age we are. One of the many tips I provide to adolescents in mindfulness class is that we can soothe ourselves with self-touch. We can rub our own arms and be aware of the feel of our hands against our limbs and of our limbs on our hands. To outsiders it simply looks as though we are cold and are trying to warm ourselves and to us, we know that we are loving ourselves, providing ourselves with the hug that we so desperately need. Another type of touch is to place our cheeks or face in our hands. If we do this with our elbow propped on a desk, it may look to others as though we are tired or bored and again, we are silently providing ourselves with the tenderness to calm our nervous system. You could hold your belly, rub your legs, give your hands a massage or sit with eyes closed, hands over your heart. What do you need? Even sitting quietly with your hands together is an example of you getting the hand holding that you need, and simply looks as though you are politely minding your own business. Yet again, nobody knows more perfectly what you need than you do. Nobody needs to know what you are doing except for you. Another technique I like to share is called the "Butterfly Hug" which involves touch and slow, methodical movement.

Free Resource: *Check out the 2-minute video example of the Butterfly Hug on YouTube from Cork Kerry Community Healthcare during their "5 Ways Over 5 Days" Series: https://www.youtube.com/watch?v=RurqWg2Bcuo or read about the butterfly hug at this site: https://emdrfoundation.org/toolkit/butterfly-hug.pdf*

Respectful, soothing touch is a gift we can give to others and respectful, soothing self-touch is a gift we can give to ourselves. It's free. It's good for you. It works.

- **Proximity:** A deer is safer being with another than on its own, and it is safer still with many deer than with one. Humans are designed to feel comforted by the presence of other mammals, including furry pets. Thankfully we can reach out through technology and remind ourselves and each other that we are not alone. Checking in on a neighbor is healthy for them and for you. Facetime and so many other incredible inventions allow us to not only speak to the people we reach to communicate with, but to see them as well.
  Snuggle your fellow mammals, hug your family or yourself, pat your dog and cuddle your cat or hamster. In fact, take refuge in a fuzzy blanket or pull out your favorite teddy bear; we're comforted by touch, including anything that feels good against our

skin. There's a reason that toddlers and small children like to hold their special blankies or pajamas – they have mammalian wisdom inside of them.

Mindful Tip: *Placing pillows around your body can be extremely supportive for your nervous system if you are experiencing feelings of loneliness, stress or anxiety*

- **Swaying Movement:** Mammals are carried inside the bodies of their mothers until they are born, and hence, are already familiar with swaying motions. Many mammals will also carry their young with them, further solidifying the sense of safety that arises from movement (kangaroos, monkeys, etc.). When an infant cries, a first instinct is often to: pick the infant up (touch), hold the infant in one's arms (proximity), make shushing sounds or sing a soft lullaby (prosocial, soothing sounds) and…to lightly sway (gentle movement). There is a part of the brain called the Cerebellum which is stimulated with rocking motion, which results in a downregulation of the rest of the brain. If you experience stress or anxiousness, or any other feeling or emotion that would be better served by regulation, consider casually swaying or rocking back and forth using a soothing rhythm that feels comfortable and nurturing for you.

Free Resource: *Check out the free videos available for multiple techniques to self-regulate at* *www.somaticexperiencing.com*

- **Sucking:** Mammals are born with the desire to suck. If a mammal does not suck, it is unlikely to survive. Hence, it is a biological design that not only preserves life, but that also serves as a calming and regulating experience for our nervous system: That is why providing an infant with a pacifier will often help them to settle – because they have received a message that their nervous system is safe. (Although, if an infant is hungry, needs to be changed, requires touch and soothing then, of course, a pacifier will not do the trick.) Some infants, toddlers, children (and some adults) will suck their thumbs in an (often) unconscious bid to calm their nervous system. (Yet another example of how brilliant the human body is.) Hence, you may find some physiological relief from anxiety or stress simply through the use of a hard candy or your favorite flavor of sucker.

Free Resource: *To learn more about what can be done to support your overall sense of well-being, and to help in your journey of reducing anxiety, please check out the information and exercises about Polyvagal Theory (an in-depth explanation of the nervous system) in this helpful and informative article (if you do not wish to read about the science* *behind Polyvagal theory, you may want to skip ahead to the part of the article titled "Examples of Polyvagal Exercises"): www.thehumancondition.com/polyvagal-theory-exercises-benefits-examples/*

As you have read, there are many "why's" when it comes to stress and anxiety. It is so important to know that *people are valid to experience stress or anxiety (or any other emotion) and they are not wrong for feeling it.* In fact, that knowledge alone can sometimes help to quash some of the stress or anxiety that people suffer from, knowing that they suffer from stress or anxiety.

Mindful Tip: *Often, when we try to figure out or justify our reason for feeling anxious, we remain stuck. We don't necessarily need to know why we feel a certain way. If we give ourselves permission to just allow the emotion to be present, then maybe we'll figure it out, or maybe it won't matter any longer. Sometimes understanding can only come once we let it go*

The few examples listed in this chapter are just the tip of the iceberg – the point of this short guide isn't to tell you everything that anyone could ever wish to know about stress or anxiety (because then it wouldn't be a simple or short guide at all), but instead to introduce you to some of the concepts of stress and anxiety so that you can mindfully become aware of what is happening for you and then select a technique that will help you to move comfortably back to feeling safe again. It is also to help you understand that feeling stressed or anxious is a normal (albeit unpleasant) experience of being human, and that there are many ways that we can befriend and overcome it. The more empowered we can become and feel with regards to handling our uncomfortable states, the less anxiety we have about feeling stressed and the less that these emotions can take over. Continue reading for more information, tips, techniques and tools for befriending and overcoming stress and anxiety.

Mindful Reflection: *Do you naturally and spontaneously cheer out loud or jump up and down when you get excited about something at work? If the answer is no, then reflect for a moment on why you will allow some emotions to control your bodily wisdom and not others…is it possible for you to access some fierce self-compassion and say to yourself, "No Stress – I love myself too much to allow you to take over today."*

Part VI: A Deeper Dive into the What

Having a definition as to what stress or anxiety are can be helpful (Reminder: They are both "a physiological state of over-activation which is unnecessary for the current situation"), but there is more to understanding stress and anxiety than just a description. We also need to know the different types.

The Three Types of Stress and Anxiety

1) Physical
2) Mental
3) Emotional

We will explore each of these branches of stress and anxiety, as well as numerous techniques for understanding, befriending, and overcoming them. Remember to honor yourself by not trying to force anything; some of these exercises may work for you and some of them may not – the goal of this guidebook is to provide a cornucopia of options so that you can create the combination that best supports you and your specific needs for the time that you need them. Also, as you read through the examples of the types of stress and anxiety, you may want to connect with which type(s) of these you tend to experience, as well as the different scenarios that may tend to put you into these states. (If reading or practicing any of these tools causes you discomfort, please consider coming back to them another time or going through them with a health professional or someone else who is able to support you.)

#1) Physical Stress or Anxiety is the body's way of alerting you to the fact that it feels unsafe. Remember, *feeling* unsafe is not the same as actually *being* unsafe. Your body's reaction to stress and anxiety is very similar to its reaction to danger and fear, which is often through the mobilization of flight or fight. As discussed earlier in the guide, symptoms of nervous symptom activation can include tight muscles and a racing heart. They can also include shallow breathing which, uncontrolled, can serve to heighten anxiety. Physical activation means that there is more energy in the body than needed; the energy doesn't match the situation, which can leave us feeling agitated, jumpy, and unable to settle. Some of the physical symptoms can include headaches, difficulty hearing people speak (because we become wired to hear threats, not talking), halitosis, chronic pain, the inability to fight off colds and infections or digestive issues, just to name a few. Basically, the body is simply a feedback mechanism, and these symptoms communicate that we need to 'take control of the wheel' and help to bring ourselves back to regulation.

Tools for calming the body when experiencing physical activation of stress or anxiety:

- Practice Self-compassion
- Get energy moving in the body (if you are feeling "ungrounded" then movement such as weights, or walking can be grounding, if you are in need of space, you may prefer yoga and if you are working off "fight" energy, you may select something like running or swimming – sometimes the best way to know what your body wants is to ask it…bodies respond when we talk to them)
- Check your blood sugar and/or stimulant intake (as mentioned earlier: caffeine, sugar, carbs, etc.)
- Investigate your hormone levels
- Ensure that you are getting enough sleep and enough deep rest – give your body what it needs

#2) Mental Stress and Anxiety is the body's way of letting you know that it has gotten caught up in ruminative thinking. It often involves an overactive and racing mind as well as time travel, either to future events (likely terrible) or events or conversations that have happened in the past. It can leave one feeling physically exhausted (due to the utilization of so much mental energy) but mentally wired. Some of the thoughts that tend to be more common to inducing stress and anxiety are thoughts surrounding something happening to you in the future or something happening to someone or something that you care about.

Tools for calming the body when experiencing mental stress or anxiety activation:

- Practice Self-compassion
- Recognize that trying to think your way out of anxiety only serves to make it worse; it's not about managing the thoughts, its about supporting the sensations. (If "not thinking" is just too difficult for you to manage, then simply recalibrate your thinking and ask yourself, "Is this a safe moment right now? What are some cues that I am safe in my environment in this moment? – there is air to breathe, there is not a fire or another life-or-death emergency, I can hear laughing in the other room, I can feel the coolness of the air conditioner on my skin…)
- Get out of your thought processes through mediums such as exercise, meditation or mindfulness
- Consider speaking to a therapist or trusted friend in order to receive help with processing your thoughts

#3) Emotional Stress or Anxiety is the body's way of letting you know that it is not currently feeling safe. It could be that it simply doesn't feel safe or that it feels unsafe (in danger). This can show up in many different ways, including feeling sensitive, or angry, irritable and easily triggered, it could feel numb, as is the case with emotional shutdown, or it could leave a person completed bewildered and confused about how they are feeling.

Tools for calming the body when experiencing emotional stress or anxiety activation:

- Practice Self-compassion
- Avoid overload by setting firm and appropriate healthy boundaries (this may include letting people know, "I just need some solitude to process what I'm going through." Give yourself space if you need it.)
- Slow down your inner world through mediums such as meditation, mindfulness or movement
- Consider speaking to a therapist or trusted friend in order to receive help with processing your emotions

The key here is to get to know your body intimately in order to discern between which form of activation you are feeling. It is possible that it could be only one type, or a combination or two or all types. The better we can become at identifying what our body is trying to tell us, the more supportive the intervention we can choose to utilize.

Mindful Tip: *Stress and anxiety are both born from a sense of danger. Curious investigation can only be done in safety, so even the act of being gently or even remotely curious as to what is happening for you instantaneously changes your relationship with your state of dysregulation*

We can employ mindfulness first by recognizing that we are in a state of suffering. Then we can look to investigate the situation a little further, "Hey, I'm feeling really anxious here – what is currently happening that could be making me feel this way?"

Familiarizing Yourself with Yourself: What are your personal bodily cues that may suggest your nervous system has been (acutely or chronically) engaged? (Place a check mark next to all that apply)

__ Feeling on-edge or restless
__ Trembling or shaking
__ Experiencing negative or turbulent thoughts
__ Uncharacteristic narcissistic behavior
__ Rash or non-future oriented decisions (that are often later regretted)
__ Difficulty concentrating/mind fog
__ Anxiety, depression, irritability, uneasy mood
__ Dilated pupils
__ Dizziness
__ Clumsiness
__ "Evil" butterflies in your stomach
__ Overly judgemental or critical of self or others
__ Uncharacteristic high pitched-voice, low-growly tone or feeling like the throat is tight or closing
__ Dry mouth

__ Halitosis (chronic bad breath)
__ Tingling
__ Eye twitch
__ Other muscle/bodily twitches
__ Hair loss not associated with aging or genetics
__ Dull or brittle hair
__ Brittle nails
__ Dry skin
__ Flushed, red or blotchy skin
__ Acne
__ Headaches
__ Clenched jaw/need for nightguard
__ Cravings
__ Difficulty hearing people when they speak even though your hearing is fine
__ Muscle tension (neck, back, shoulders, legs)
__ Rapid heartbeat or heart palpitations
__ Quick, shallow breathing
__ High cholesterol
__ High blood pressure
__ Infection (cold sore, yeast infection, canker sore)
__ Autoimmune flair-ups (psoriasis, lupus, eczema, fibromyalgia, irritable bowel syndrome, allergies, etc.)
__ Delayed tissue repair (long time for cuts/bruises to heal)
__ Cold/flu
__ Constipation
__ Diarrhea
__ Indigestion, gas, or bloating

__ Anemia or other mineral or vitamin deficiencies
__ Sweating (palms, underarms, head)
__ Decreased libido
__ Hormone production issues
__ Insomnia
__ Oversleeping
__ Racing thoughts
__ An unnecessary sense of urgency
__ Picking at or biting nails, picking at acne, pulling hair, or other unconscious habits
__ Constantly fidgeting or moving
__ Addiction or dependency issue(s) (drugs, alcohol, overworking, social media, shopping, sex, fawning, overexercising, perfectionism, etc.)

Mindful Tip: *Any type of nervous system activation may result in a craving for foods containing sugar, such as sweets or carbohydrates. From an evolutionary perspective, our bodies were biologically designed to crave sweet things as we were 'pre-wired' to build fat stores during times of plenty (spring and summer months) in order to prepare for famine (winter months). When we consume foods that are sweet, it communicates a message of safety and security to our brain*

These are just a few of the ways that our bodies will try to communicate with us that something needs to be addressed in order to for us to return to homeostasis, where optimal health and wellbeing reside. Nervous system activation shows up in different combinations for everyone and it can be extremely helpful to know what your personal signs are. For example, I know that I have been activated when my heart is pounding, I have the desire to act immediately (respond to the email or make that comment *right now*) or when I realize that my quad muscles have suddenly tightened. For my partner, his telltale sign is hands that are burning hot, and my daughter's pupils will dilate to saucers if she is anxious about an upcoming exam at school. Those are all immediate reactions to stress, but more chronic (long-term) symptoms in our family are that my husband needs his mouth guard due to night-time jaw clenching, I become anemic, my daughter will break out in acne, and my son will get eczema (skin is sometimes referred to as a "magic mirror," as it may reflect on the outside when there is dysregulation occurring on the inside). A friend of mine gets an eye twitch and a couple of friends of mine will experience canker sores or cold sores, while another will experience heart palpitations. The longer that we go ignoring our bodily symptoms, the louder they will get – eventually resorting to disease or worse if they need to. Both Dr. Gabor Mate in his book *When the Body Says No* and Dr. Bessel van der Kolk in his book *The Body Keeps the Score* discuss at length some of the long-term implications of not recognizing and responding to bodily cues. To suppress our feelings, thoughts or emotions is to suppress our nervous system. The more mindful we become at detecting these issues as they arise, the more empowered we are to take the steps to support our nervous system and practice self-care.

Mindful Tip: *Bring awareness to your cravings, as they may be an indicator of what is happening for you internally. For example, craving "comfort foods" may indicate that you are not currently regulated (and hence, need to be "comforted"). If you are in the "up" position of your seesaw (sympathetic activation), you may crave alcohol, cigarettes or other foods or activities in your body's attempt to "bring you down" through the process of downregulation. Similarly, if you are in the "down" position of your teeter-totter (dorsal parasympathetic activation), you may crave such things as sugar, carbs, caffeine or other stimulants such as watching a horror movie in order to "lift you up" via upregulation*

Mindful Exercise: Straw Breathing

One of the many ways that we can communicate to our nervous system (and amygdala) that we are safe is to increase our exhalation time so that it is longer than our inhalation. As discussed previously, when we are stressed or anxious, one of the ways that our body will respond is by quickening our breathing with rapid, shallow breaths. When we consciously take a long, slow, deep inhale and follow it with an even longer exhale we basically "override" the system that is trying to control the body. Breathing in this way provides more oxygen to the brain, which opens up accessibility for greater clarity.

- Take a nice and comfortable long, slow, deep breath through your nose

- For a longer duration than the inhale (preferably twice as long if that is comfortable for you), let that breath out through pursed lips as though you are blowing the air through a straw, relaxing your body as you do

That's it! There are plenty of examples on YouTube, however I have found that some of the clips have breathing that is too fast, which ends up actually eliciting a stressed or anxious response. Find a pace that is almost exaggerated on the exhalation, yet still comfortable – if you feel relaxed when it is over, you're doing it right. If you find that your body does not feel better, continue to experiment with it – if the breathing count doesn't work, change it. If the thought of breathing through a straw doesn't resonate for you, imagine that you are playing a flute on the exhalation instead. Do whatever you need to in order to support your body best.

> **Mindful Tip:** *If you find yourself saying something like, "I'm doing my daily affirmations but I'm still crawling out of my skin!" then it is time to change to a different modality for shifting yourself back to regulation. Just because something has worked in the past does not necessarily mean that it will work in the future and just because something has not worked in the past does not mean that it won't work now. Just as your mood shifts, so too do your wants and needs*

Or if you prefer, try this little trick that you likely didn't even know that your body already knew:

Mindful Exercise: Indulge in a Sigh

Have you ever had someone ask you, "What's the matter?" because you unconsciously let out a big sigh? That's the genius of your body at work! Basically, your body is forcing its own version of "Straw Breathing" in an attempt to help you to calm your nervous system and return to a more optimal state. Reflect for a moment where you are or what you are doing when you sigh: at work, finally arriving at your destination, right after somebody you care about says something upsetting to you, after looking at your never-ending to-do list, etc. – what all of these examples have in common is that your unconscious sigh occurs *after* a stressful event has occurred (even a mini-stressful event), in order to automatically release some of the mobilized energy that had been created in the nervous system. A sigh includes a deep breath, a comforting (mammalian technique) sound, and muscle relaxation. It's your body's own way of telling your brain, "It's okay, you are safe now. You can relax." The cool part is that you can communicate that to your system anytime you want or need to. Try as you might, it is pretty difficult to remain anxious after letting out a few good sighs:

- Take a big inhalation

- Indulge in a big, long exhalation as you make a sighing noise that is as loud and as long as you want it to be, while allowing your muscles to soften and relax (you may even choose to enjoy "rag doll" – an over-exaggeration of allowing the body to go limp)

-

- Repeat often (Okay, that part isn't necessary, but remember that the more often that you show your body what it feels like to be safe, the better your body gets at: 1) automatically noticing when you are out of balance, and 2) bringing itself back to homeostasis)

An Example of Nervous System Activations

Recently, while I was working on this book, my husband Keith went out for a bike ride on his own. While making his way up one of the nearby hills, a dog that has escaped from the back yard where it was normally housed came charging directly at him, viciously ready to attack. Instantaneously, Keith's amygdala detected the threat and activated his sympathetic nervous system in order to ensure his survival. Because he was climbing a hill on the bike, flight was not an option – the dog would be too fast for him. Activated for the 'fight' response, Keith instantly unclipped from his pedals and held his bike as a bodily shield while he stood his ground against the out-of-control animal. The dog was snarling loudly, his teeth bared as he ferociously lunged at Keith again and again in an attempt to bite him. At each lunge Keith used both hands to force his bike out in front of him in an attempt to hold the animal at bay. There was no doubt, the dog was out of control and not going to give up: Without intervention, this was going to be a very long fight. A good Samaritan driver arrived on the scene and immediately upon seeing what was happening, drove his car towards the dog while loudly honking his horn. The dog was relentless and Keith and the driver worked together, one using a bike and the other a vehicle and a horn to deter the animal. By the time the owner heard the commotion, traffic was stopped on both sides of the road as the dog tried numerous paths of attack to get around the car and bike in order to get to Keith. Once the dog was secured, the hero driver jumped out of his car to ask Keith if he was okay and the owner of the dog ran back out to apologize. The proximity and concern from those two men provided coregulation for Keith's activated and mobilized nervous system. Biking the rest of the way home required Keith to utilize his muscles, expelling the excess energy that had been provided to him in order to survive the emergency. The fact that he biked *away* from the event would have allowed Keith's system to register that 'flight' was now being accessed, effectively closing the circuit of activation. By the time that Keith arrived home and told me the story, his upregulated nervous system was already back to homeostasis and he was completely calm as he told me about what happened. (*Important to note: If Keith had spent the rest of the ride home rehashing what had happened or thinking angry thoughts about the dog or his owner, that would have kept his body mobilized with fight or flight activation and he would have likely come home angry and agitated.)

However…

Through the magic of mirror neurons, Keith's telling of the story alone activated my nervous system. As he had spoken, I had pictured him going through this horrific ordeal, and my mind continuously flashed to thoughts of him being in danger and of what could have happened. That evening, while Keith slept like a baby beside me in bed, I was sleepless. Although I was calm (emotionally regulated) knowing that he was safe now, and my thoughts were those of gratitude (mentally regulated) for so many things, including that unnamed hero, my body felt like I had just consumed ten pots of coffee (physically dysregulated). My skin was buzzing, my heart was pounding, my body had various and consistent twitches and I could feel the thickness of the blood coursing through my veins. Now, 90% of the time slow, deep breathing and calming thoughts help me to settle my nervous system, but not this time. Finally, I asked my body what it needed from me, as I just wasn't able to make my way back to regulation through my regular channels and techniques. Immediately I had a craving to don my workout clothes and go for a run in the middle of the night; a long, exhausting run. "Aha!" Of course, how could I not have thought of that? Deep breathing isn't going to help the physical activation present in my body; after hearing Keith's story, my mirror neurons picked up on the danger and wanted me to flee! Laying in bed with my eyes closed, I imaged running along a route that Keith and I used to jog before we moved. I immersed myself in the sound of the gravel under my shoes, the feeling of the impact of my feet hitting the ground and lifting, hitting the ground and lifting…I remembered the sensation of the burn of exertion ripping through my lungs. Instantaneously my body relaxed; I simply had to support it in the way that it needed to be supported. (Remember that the mind doesn't know the difference between something happening versus *thinking* that something is happening, which is why our thoughts can easily and instantly "stress us out." In this case, I simply used my thoughts and imagination to *calm* me instead.) I fell asleep after promising myself that the first order of business for the next morning was to get some exercise in order to blow out any remaining unexpressed energy.

The point of this example is…

- The sympathetic nervous system worked exactly as it should have; the amygdala sensed a threat and took charge of the brain – flight/fight response was activated, mobilizing Keith with a burst of energy in the form of heightened senses and increased oxygen and strength to muscles. (There were many other physiological changes, too many to name, but shrinkage of the feet in order to make him nimbler as well as thickening of the blood so that he didn't bleed out in the event that he was injured are just a couple more examples of the miracle of the body)
- Keith was able to literally play out the 'fight' (and then subsequently 'flight') response – the activation kept him safe

- Coregulation works, even if it offered from regulated strangers
- Expelling remaining mobilized energy (riding home) plays a huge role in calming physiology
- Mirror neurons work; even *hearing* the story sent my amygdala into alarm status (what are some things that you are exposed to that set off your nervous system; the news, social media posts, scary movies, violent music, who-done-it murder/mystery books…)
- Physiology does speak to us; what are your thoughts, flashes, insights, hunches, cravings, dreams trying to communicate to you?
- It was only upon getting home that Keith realized that he had injured his ankle, presumably from having to quickly unclip from his pedals and jump behind his bike. The rush of adrenaline that had kicked in during his sympathetic activation had done its two major jobs: 1) Given Keith a burst of energy which he was able to utilize in his "fight" with the dog as well as, 2) Dulling his bodily pain sensors so that he was not distracted or slowed by pain during battle

Basically, the point here is that activation is not our enemy; it is here to save us. When we understand what is happening when our body moves into dysregulation and how to get it back, we can befriend and overcome the stresses and anxieties of everyday life.

Free Resource: *One of my favorite experts in the field of stress and anxiety is Dr. Kimberley Quinlan. Check out her podcast for her accessible and down-to-earth explanations and advice: Your Anxiety Toolkit*

Part VII: The How

"See if you can give yourself gifts that may be true blessings, such as self-acceptance, or some time each day with no purpose. Practice feeling deserving enough to accept these gifts without obligation – to simply receive from yourself, and from the universe."

– Jon Kabat-Zinn

It is often when we most need to nourish our bodies that we don't. It is when we are faced with anxiety, or stress, or panic, or fear, or anger or tumultuous world events that we most need to take care of ourselves and yet, that is when we put it on the back burner. You are important. Your health is important. Your wellbeing is important. If you are reading this book right now, then you are doing it because you know that these things are true. So, let's take a look at ways to support you in your relationship of befriending and overcoming anxiety.

Basically, there are two things that need to happen to change a relationship with stress or anxiety:

1) They need to be interrupted when they occur (plain and simple – we need to stop strengthening our memorized habits of anxious thoughts, stressful feelings and anxiety-provoking sensations)

2) The brain needs to be rewired so that stress and anxiety are not the first or dominant neural pathways (the brain needs to be introduced to, and learn new ways of thinking, new "default modes")

When creating your toolkit there are a coupe of points that need to be covered that have not yet been touched upon. The first one is the importance of non-judgement: Years ago, when I was still holding individual sessions, I was working with an adolescent that was in dire need of improving her levels of self-acceptance and self-love. She had created some statements that felt very supportive and loving for her to tell herself, and when it came time for her to close her eyes and actually think them, she couldn't do it. After a moment her beautiful blue eyes flew open and when I queried, "What happened?" she replied, "I can't." When I asked her why not, she responded, "Because I would be so embarrassed if anyone ever knew that I was saying these things to myself."

Create a boundary of acceptance where you are protected and free from the judgement of others and the judgement of self. Feeling judged, whether it is the judgements of other people or self-judgement alerts the amygdala to danger and restricts our ability to think clearly and live optimally. If some of the suggestions in this guide seem silly to you but they work nonetheless, then it is nobody's business to judge; you don't even have to let other people know. Who cares if you give yourself a hug in the bathroom stall at work, or if you practice straw breathing while you're driving in the car to work? Whose business is it if you silently tell yourself that you are important and loved while you wait for your turn at the checkout, hum loudly in the shower or hug your teddy bear at night? It is your business and your business alone, and if it works and doesn't cause harm to anyone, then who cares? Heck, just this morning I looked at my reflection in the mirror and smiled as I thought, "I really like you. You're not perfect (implied with humour, *'not even close'*), but you sure do try hard at anything you do (implied with appreciation, *'and I really admire that about you'*)" (and believe me, you would laugh your head off if you could hear the pep talks I silently give myself during a challenging hike or workout!). It is easy to get caught up in our evolutionary concern of wanting to be cast in a positive light in the eyes of others, but we know now that we don't have to live that way. What works for you in your relationship to befriend and overcome stress and anxiety is what works for you in your relationship to befriend and overcome stress and anxiety. Period.

Mindful Tip: *Imagine that each thought or action that you take to offer yourself soothing, self-compassion or a sense of safety creates a new neural pathway in your brain*

The second point is about Medication. Full disclosure; on a personal level medication is often not my first resort, nor is it necessarily my favorite; I prefer not to take it if I don't have to. But if I *do* need to take it for something, then I do. If you are like me, you may be medication hesitant. I respect that, and would like to offer you a simple question: *How do you train your body to memorize feeling safe if your body no longer remembers how?* Because of the stigma that can sometimes surround mental health issues, many people hesitate to get help, and by the time they do, it is possible that they no longer remember what it feels like to feel grounded or connected. What if you are someone who has been so anxious or stressed, for so long, that the plasticity of your brain has memorized feeling chronically stressed or anxious or even chronically panicked? Then in my humble (and completely non-medical) opinion, a prescription for mood stabilizing medication from your health provider may be the place for you and your body to start. All of these options don't work if they don't work – and if you cannot find a place or even sense of calm, then it sounds like the next order of business may be to see your doctor.

Free Resource: *Often stress and anxiety can be related to our unconsciously learned attachment styles which stem from childhood. To learn more about yourself, including communication styles and unconscious beliefs, take the quiz on attachment styles at www.dianepooleheller.com*

More Techniques for Interrupting Stress or Anxiety When They Occur:

Neural Linguistic Programming

NLP for short, Neural Linguistic Programming is a fancy word that translated to normal language means Brain (Neural) Language (Linguistic) Programming. Basically, it is a psychological approach that utilizes different ways of communicating with ourselves, such as thoughts, language, pictures, and patterns of behaviour learned through experience to specific and desired outcomes: We can train our brain using different techniques to quickly respond in a way we want them to. For example, I had mentioned previously that when I start to lose my cool after being triggered by my daughter being late, I think to myself, STOP, STOP, STOP! My automatic reaction upon thinking those words is to indeed, **S**top, **T**ake a few breaths, **O**bserve my internal reactions and external environment and then **P**roceed in a better manner than the track I'm currently on. NLP at work. Now, you may be wondering how this is different from The STOP Practice that was discussed earlier in the guide. The difference is that I am not using this as a mindfulness practice; I have programmed it into my brain that as soon as I yell "STOP" in my head I completely and immediately release whatever I am saying or doing, right in the middle of saying or doing it (yes, mid-sentence) and then I immediately and automatically slow and deepen my breathing. I literally STOP. (It reminds me of a girlfriend of mine from high school; her dad had somehow rigged her car so that if she hit 80km per hour the car would automatically shift into neutral; saying STOP to myself immediately shifts me from speeding into neutral.) I've also used the technique for when I begin to get anxious about water leakage (I know, I know…we all have our own strange triggers). As soon as I become aware of the fact that I am getting tangled up into anxious rumination or stressful thoughts, then I STOP and picture a rabbit hole. It works to immediately break that train of thought. The rabbit hole in my mind's eye signifies (not too surprisingly) "Don't go down that rabbit hole again!" I already know that rabbit holes lead to nowhere good, so I imagine seeing the rabbit hole in the ground and deciding not to go down it. It took some time to get there, as I had to practice finding something, *anything* else to think about in order to distract me from that memorized thought pattern, but it works for me. Every. Single. Time. No joke. Now, there are times when a moment later the thought will rear its ugly head again, "No, seriously Alex, but what will we *do* if there was a leak right now? How would you contain the water?" (Yes, I realize that this particular anxious fear sounds ridiculous, but I'm just being honest with you.) If that happens, I immediately picture the rabbit hole again and think something along the lines of, "Nice try; I'm not going down there no matter how much you try to entice me." And by the second attempt, the anxiety dissipates and I go about my business.

In order to fully maximize NLP, what you want to do is figure out which modality you prefer. For example, when you think, what words do you use to describe your thoughts? For example, do you think, "Hmm…that <u>smells</u> fishy," or "That <u>sounds</u> like it might be off to me," or "That <u>looks</u> like something

I don't want to get involved with," "That doesn't <u>feel</u> right," or "That is really putting a bad <u>taste</u> in my mouth"? Deciphering this may help you find your modality preference: sight, sound, taste, touch or feel. For me, I prefer several of them, using STOP for certain triggers, the rabbit hole for spiraling thoughts, and my gut reaction and other physical sensations for other issues. Let's say that social media makes you stressed or anxious (which it is clinically proven to do, so you may want to seriously consider limiting your exposure if possible): You may choose to program your brain to interrupt negative thought programs through imagining that you *smell* garbage when you feel yourself getting upset over a post, or you may program your brain to *hear* alarm bells, signalling a "sounding of the alarm" that it's time to do other things, or memorize the *taste* of liver or a half-chewed multi-vitamin (not the tasty kind) to remind you that proceeding will leave a nasty taste in your mouth, or a *picture* of a sign that says "Caution: Landslide Area" to remind you that you don't want to get carried away, or imagine that you are *feeling* a burn on your fingertips to remind you not to do anything that's going to get you burned.

> **<u>Mindful Tip:</u>** *If you are an animal-lover, you may want to use the word "Sit!" for your NLP trigger, imagining that your stress or anxiety is like a dog that needs to just stop barking and running around, and can trust that you are in charge*

Tapping

This variation of thought interruption comes in many forms. (Some people use an elastic around their wrist and snap it in order to cause minor physical discomfort and act as a reminder to get out of their head and into their body.) Tapping can be used as an intervention for anxious-thought interruption, or stress reduction, as well as a tool to promote grounding, and to rewire and reprogram the brain.

"Bodily Tapping" consists of gentle tapping off body parts in order to get a sense of the body and to stimulate the skin. This may be especially helpful for people who tend to feel disembodied (downregulated) or struggle with clumsiness.

A very general overview of "EFT (Emotional Freedom Techniques) Tapping" involves saying or thinking what you are anxious about while gently tapping your fingers (as if you were tapping them on the table) at different energy meridians on your body, such as the fleshy side of the hand just below the pinky fingers, the temples, above the nose where eyebrows begin and just below the clavicles. Tapping generally takes a few rounds, and the statements shift from stating the source of the stress or anxiety to statements that progressively get more positive in nature, such as moving from "I am anxious about my health" to "I am looking forward to feeling confident in my health" and then (if it feels comfortable and authentic), "I am grateful for my good health." As with all of these tools, it's all about finding what fits and feels good for you, including the comments that you say to yourself.

Free Resources: *You can find more information on EFT Tapping at Nick Ortner's website: www.thetappingsolution.com. Should this be something that you would like to try, there is also a free downloadable app available for you phone*

Thinking New Thoughts

We now know that because of The Negativity Bias that humans have a propensity towards negative thoughts. In fact the majority of most people's thoughts are negative even though most of our daily experiences are either neutral or positive. Not only that, but the large majority of the thoughts that we have today are the same thoughts that we had yesterday (wash our hair the same way in the shower, brush our teeth the same way, drive the same route to work…). Another miracle fact about our brains is that they will create "shortcuts" (memorized neural pathways) for the thoughts and actions that we regularly do in order to provide more mental and energetic resources for other actions: This is why we can drive home, but not remember how we did or, or walk away from the house and not recall if we turned off the stove – which of course, we did. Our brains memorize and create "default" thoughts and actions based on what we've done in the past – kind of like how YouTube figures out your preferences and then suggests more of the same. This tool is beneficial if our memorized thoughts, feelings and emotions are normally neutral or positive, but not so great when we've trained our minds and bodies how to be stressed or anxious. A way to change that? Think new thoughts: As many and as often as you can. I'm speaking from personal experience when I tell you that this is a lot more challenging that it sounds. What you want to do is think thoughts that you have never thought before in your life in order to create new neural pathways (connections in our brain that influence thinking and belief patterns). These thoughts don't have to be about anything in particular, they just have to be brand new. Imagine that every single time you think a new thought, and really pause to consider it, that your brain gets bigger and smarter. In essence, that's what happens. Not only that, but you create new pathways from which your thoughts and belief systems (and thought habits) can now arise.

> **Free Resource:** *To access some "new thoughts" that you may find beneficial, such as "Would you let your anxiety go if you could?" check out The Sedona Method, which has helped countless people to liberate themselves from their memorized emotion and thought patterns: The Sedona Method channel on YouTube, The Sedona Method podcast 'Letting Go' with Hale Dwoskin or www.sedona.com*

The only caveat here is that the thoughts need to be neutral or positive; no purposely selecting negative thoughts to dwell on. Although this may seem like an obvious guideline, for anyone who has spent a lifetime diligently being on the lookout for the negative, breaking free of old habits can be hard. When I first started this many years ago (simply because I really liked the concept of creating a "new" brain by thinking new thoughts), I really had to search for thoughts that were new. When a class that I was teaching at a Middle School asked me what my new thought for that day was, I replied that it had been, "I could wear a dress or skirt to class today." They all looked at me like I had three heads because the thought was crazy; normally I wore jeans. Well, it was a new thought and it counted. Now my thoughts come so much more effortlessly; they are much deeper, and rich with creativity. I have a new, much less anxious or stressed brain.

For more science behind the importance of thinking neutral or positive thoughts versus negative ones, we will once again return back to the metaphor of the seesaw: If the amygdala is represented with the "high" and the "low", and the pre-frontal cortex is represented by being in balance, there is another part of the brain called the anterior cingulate that works as the fulcrum in the middle that supports the seesaw's ability to balance. Negativity (especially anger, but stress and anxiety as well) is like a corrosive material that eats away at, and undermines the effectiveness of the fulcrum (the anterior cingulate) - too much of it and now the teeter-totter is off balance and becomes more susceptible to being stuck in the up or down, changing and influencing the way we see the world and the way we behave. For example, you may have noticed that without some type of intervention (personal or otherwise), generally speaking, over time angry people become angrier, depressed people become more depressed and yes, anxious or stressed people become more anxious or stressed. (The anterior cingulate is also impeded by anything that increases inflammation, including improper diet and lack of sleep.) The good news is that this doesn't have to be the case. Just like riding a bike, the old saying of, "Where you look is where you go" holds true with our emotional and cognitive state. Any and all of the tools, techniques and practices in this book will help to keep your brain (including your pre-frontal cortex and anterior cingulate) healthier.

> **Mindful Tip:** *When you notice that you have become activated and are feeling stressed or anxious, shift your perspective by considering, "Oh wow; look at how much you care about this!"*

Practicing a Feeling of Safety

"Consciously holding onto a feeling is better than feeling like a feeling is holding onto you."

– Hale Dwoskin

Many of us have practiced, if not perfected, the sense of feeling unsafe. Reprogram your neural circuitry by practicing (and hopefully perfecting) the sense of being safe. There are unlimited ways to do this, including:

1. Think back to a time in your life when you felt safe. Connect with that feeling; what were your thoughts? What were your feelings? What were the sensations in your body? Take your time to

marinate in the memory, and allow it to soak into your nervous system

2. Catch yourself in a moment of safety. This might be while you are comfortably laying in bed, lazily enjoying a cup of coffee, or enjoying a sunset. Connect with the sensations in your body. How does it *feel* to feel safe? Extend and linger in that moment, and the awareness of safety for as long as you can.

Remembering Dr. Rick Hanson's quote from earlier, "The brain is like Velcro for the negative and Teflon for the positive," we want to switch that around and teach our brains to be like Velcro for the positive (feeling safe). That is done through lingering in the moment and really "locking" that thought, memory or sensation into place. (We can also train our brains to be like Teflon for the negative by not allowing ourselves to dwell on negativity or ruminating thought processes – when I notice that I'm thinking something that is unnecessary and negative, I say to myself, "Negativity bores me. This bores me," or I imagine that it is a hot potato and I want to drop it as soon as possible.)

Vocalizing and Other Out-Breath Techniques

We already touched upon the benefits of creating sounds that resonate with your energy level (one of the multiple mammalian comfort techniques), but the nervous system benefits extend beyond just that. Anything that we do that extends the outbreath supports optimal functioning of the nervous system by communicating to the brain that the body is safe. This means that *singing* is good for reducing anxiety, as is *playing a wind instrument* or *blowing bubbles* in the backyard or at the park. In fact, even painting your nails and blowing them dry does the same thing! Who knew that stress and anxiety reduction could be so much fun?

Playing

Simply the act of "playing" is incredible for reducing anxiety. While competitive games can be activating (and are not necessarily recommended for stress reduction), just "playing" is a wonderful deactivator. If you have children in your life, consider playing Hot Wheels or My Little Pony with them. Kids or not, roll in the grass, play on the swings, skip on your way to the mailbox, play on a floatie in the water, jump on a trampoline, or wrestle with your dog. Find one of those little wooden paddle things with a ball attached to it via an elastic and see how many times in a row you can hit it. Be a kid again! "Playing" reinforces to our body and mind that we are safe, because no animal will play when it is in danger; it's a complete reinforcement to the bodily unit that all is well. ("Playing" as a stress or anxiety-reduction technique has been clinically researched and proven to work – this is not just a silly recommendation; it is a tried, tested and true method of nervous system regulation and an excellent tool for maintaining or achieving homeostasis in the body and mind.)

<u>Mindful Reminder:</u> *We can even create some playfulness in our thoughts: Becoming stressed or anxious about being stressed or anxious simply reinforces the neural pathways for stress and anxiety. Instead of allowing your body to respond to things as though they are a three-alarm fire, relax: Invite a mindful, compassionate and playful relationship with your habituated response pattern. "Hello Stress – I'm heading to the store now and have lots to do, but you're welcome to come with me if you like." Allowing the emotion to be present without getting caught up in it teaches your nervous system that you do not need to respond to every moment of activation with alarm. This type of kind and open acceptance allows for you – not the emotion – to be in charge*

Practicing Restorative or Hatha Yoga

Yoga, specifically Restorative and/or Hatha Yoga are a type of yoga that is done with the intention of reconnecting and coming back to oneself; to offer rest and restoration to the body. In restorative or hatha yoga, the goal is not to 'get' somewhere, the invitation is to relinquish any type of "doing" or the desire to "get it right" or be perfect. The poses in these types of yoga are longer than those in conventional yoga, which allows for a physiological shift that results in mental rest. Restorative and hatha yoga both invite the ego to *not* interact with stimulus, which helps to support and strengthen the relationship between body and mind.

These types of yoga are also excellent ways to practice mindfulness, and the movement may be especially supportive for individuals who find that lack of motion activates their sympathetic nervous system.

> **<u>Mindful Tip:</u>** *It takes a lot of energy to be stressed or anxious, which can leave a person feeling mentally, emotionally or physically exhausted. If you find that you are ever "too tired to rest," then instead of using distraction as your first line of defense, consider putting yourself into a restorative position of relaxation through the use of a weighted eye mask, reduced sound and light, and a supportive position for your body. If it would be comfortable for you, consider using pillows or blankets to cradle, wrap or weight your body while you focus on the feelings of safety and comfort. Familiarize yourself with the taste of relaxation. You may also choose to listen to calm, soothing music or sounds or to utilize aromatherapy scents that are calming for you. When the body senses a lack of muscular engagement, the mind picks up on the fact that there is nothing for it to do, and it allows your nervous system to relax*

Purposely Engaging in Pleasant Thoughts

We're not playing Pollyanna here – this is never about pretending that you are happy when you are not. If you are unhappy then choose another tool, such as giving yourself permission to enjoy a good cry, or Name it to Tame it, or calling a supportive friend or therapist, or practicing some self-compassion and taking the night off from "doing." But if you're not unhappy, and in you're in the space to do so, try consciously selecting thoughts that make you feel good. This is all about rewiring your brain so that when it runs on autopilot the autopilot is set to drift towards pleasant thoughts versus anxious or unpleasant ones. That's all. This is science, pure and simple.

Here are some suggestions for pleasant thoughts (consider using these as meditations or mindfulness exercises, or merely as places for your mind to wander):

1. Pleasant, loving, funny, or silly memories that make you smile, laugh, or simply feel good

2. Imagining your best day. There are no limits for this one; money, time, location, etc. do not come into play here – the sky is the limit.

3. Creating a dream job in your mind (I always wanted to travel the world as a National Geographic photographer or be the best goalie in the NHL – it doesn't matter that I'm terrible at taking pictures and that I'm not good at skating)

4. Favorite vacation spots (whether you've been there or not)

5. Reminiscing on moments that you were proud of yourself, felt special, felt loved, felt safe, felt wonderful, etc. (my husband still loves to tell me how proud he was in his bit-part role of a "crew-cut angel" during his fourth-grade class play…it makes him smile every time)

6. Anything at all that you can think of, real or imagined, that promotes only positive feelings and emotions for you. (Remember, you are flexing the muscles in your brain to become stronger at defaulting to thoughts and sensations that are pleasant and safe)

*If these things seem silly or trivial to you, reflect for a moment on where your mind normally goes when it wanders; finances, relationships, work, past hurts, current world events, future worries… Thoughts that are left to run unsupervised and amok are the thoughts that continue to program and wire our brains, and continue to shape the perception and reality of our lives. If you are not happy with your current reality, you can change the view by monitoring and directing your thoughts. If you're going to be thinking something anyway, why not consciously choose for it to be a thought that is supportive and beneficial for your overall health and wellbeing versus something that undermines and erodes your overall health and wellbeing?

Indulging in Calm and Soothing Environments

The goal of a lot of these practices is to soak them into your DNA, to allow them to strengthen the neural pathways of safety, and help to dislodge, diminish and weaken the neural pathways that lead to anxiety and other negative states of mind. When you indulge (mindfully savor) calm and soothing environments, you work to do just that. If you enjoy having baths or showers, then truly feel what it's like to pamper yourself in the warmth of the water. Become immersed in the serenity of lying on the grass and looking up at the trees or the sky, be aware of the sense of relief and comfort as you lay down on the couch or in your bed or sit by the ocean and truly feel your body relax as you watch the waves gently lap against the shore. One of my favorite times is when my husband takes the kids out for a while and I get to just sit cross legged on the couch in the silence of an empty home. Where do you go already, or where can you go that will elicit a response of feeling peaceful? It could be that the morning train, with its methodical movement is your safe-haven, or the bubble of your car during the morning or afternoon commute when you have the opportunity to listen to your favorite music. Perhaps it is a local coffee shop or the garden in your yard. It could be anywhere at all, and the way to wire the benefits into your being is through the use of mindful awareness in feeling settled.

> **Mindful Tip:** *Anytime you notice a thought popping up that stops you from being in the present moment, ask yourself, "How does that feel in my body right now?" You may begin to notice that even one seemingly "insignificant and tiny" thought can produce a very powerful reaction. Breathe into any part of your body that feels tense and invite for it to relax. Practicing this regularly will enhance your ability to detect and change negative thought patterns before they get a chance to take root and grow*

Getting a Good Therapist

As mentioned previously, there are so many different modalities for therapy. Finding a therapist that you feel comfortable and safe with (and preferably like as well) doesn't always happen right off the bat. If you tried out a certain type of therapy that doesn't work for you, or met with a specialist that you didn't resonate with, keep looking; sometimes it's like dating – you need to play the field before settling down.

There is nothing weak about seeking professional help, nor is it ever anything to be embarrassed about. It truly takes a lot of courage to take steps to change your life. To be authentically seen and heard by another, perhaps for the first time one's life, can be an act of bravery. So often, even the mere act of being non-judgementally witnessed or having one's experience or reality acknowledged can be an incredibly powerful tool for reducing stress and anxiety.

Giving Yourself Some Credit

Clearly, you've done something right in your life. You wouldn't have made it this far if you haven't. Take some time to honestly recognize what you have accomplished. Whether it was obtaining your PhD or getting out of bed this morning, it doesn't matter; what matters is that there is something for you to acknowledge that you've done right. Celebrate mastery as often as you can, not because it feeds your ego but because it reinforces to your brain that you are making progress. We don't build self-confidence by being told that we're great, we build it by making our way through something that required effort or was challenging for us, and then knowing that we succeeded. Were you able to have *one less* anxious thought today? So many of us (too many of us) spend a lifetime telling ourselves what we have done and what we are doing (and what we might do) that's wrong; it is time to rewrite those old programs that clearly are not working for us and to acknowledge all of the things that are right.

Finding the Right Fit

As mentioned previously, take these tools for a test drive and see what works for you: Different moods and variations of stress require different interventions. For example, if the activation you are experiencing is your 'seesaw' in the 'up' position, you may find it very helpful to softly and gently rub down your arms, much like patting a cat. However, if the activation you are experiencing is your 'seesaw' in the 'down' position, you will likely find it much more helpful to rub up your arms (like rustling the cat's fur in the wrong position). One modality (the former) supports downregulation of the nervous system (bringing you *down* to neutral) whereas the other modality (the latter) supports upregulation of the nervous system (bringing you *up* to neutral). Find the right fit and practice self-compassion as you dismiss anything that is not personally helpful.

Creating Healthy Boundaries

Just as children who do not have healthy boundaries suffer from anxiety, so do we adults. In fact, one can experience a significant drop in overall stress simply by defining and adopting strong and supportive boundaries. This can include the boundaries that we have for others regarding their treatment of us, as well as the boundaries that we have for ourselves in our treatment of us. Personal boundaries are just that: Personal. Get to know yourself on a deeper level as you discover what is important to you; what you will accept or tolerate and what you will not. This may include things like whether or not you respond to work emails during your time away from the office, what type of tone you will accept from people in your life, and other important issues such as ensuring that you schedule self-care, and then protecting that time. You may find that journaling, researching boundary-setting (there is lots of useful free information on the internet), or speaking with someone who has strong boundaries may be helpful for you.

Mindful Reminder: *Stress and anxiety are simply signposts that something is wrong; a state of being that let's us know that something's off, and needs to be addressed. It may be that the item needing to be addressed is that you are in need of more self-care. Dysregulated states want us to move back to regulation*

Rewiring Negative Thought Patterns

The most common self-critical thoughts consist of feeling as though who one is, is not enough, that what one has is not enough, or that what one does is not enough. Reflect for a moment and check in to see if any of those thoughts ring true for you. If not, what are your thoughts or belief patterns, and in which ways are they unsupportive for you? These thoughts can produce a host of challenging emotions, not the least of which are stress anxiety (along with guilt, shame, depression and resentment). Instead of reinforcing thoughts or beliefs that do not serve you, create *new* thoughts to take their place. If you are going to have the thoughts anyway, why not just adjust them a little so that they support your well-being versus destabilize it? The list of thoughts and affirmations that you can reprogram with is endless, but here are some suggestions to help get you started:

- Who I am is enough

- What I do is enough

- What I have is enough

- I can only do what I can do, and I can not do more than that

- I lovingly honor that 'doing my best' means 'doing the best that I can in this moment with how I am feeling'

- I am human and I am experiencing what it is like to be human in this moment

- I give myself permission to be kind to me

- I love myself

Personally, I also find quotes and phrases incredibly helpful as reminders, and as support systems for gently swaying my mind into a different direction. I wrote a quick handbook on meditation called, *Breath. Relax. Release: A Simple Guide to Meditation and Mindfulness* because I was inspired to do so after creating a couple of tent cards for my kitchen and bedroom that reminded me to "Breathe. Relax. Release." (The short guidebook includes about a dozen of my favorite meditations and is available on Amazon for approximately $10 Canadian.)

Free Resource: *Sign up for free daily or weekly quotes and inspiring messages at projecthappiness.org*

Practicing Mindfulness

Mindfulness is the act of being non-judgementally open and aware, with a sense of kindness, to the present moment. It involves being fully aware of the moment that you are in without creating a story around what is happening. To mindfully eat an apple is to be aware of the feeling of the apple in your hand, the muscles that are being utilized in your hand to hold it, as well as the movements required to chew, while also being aware of the crispness and taste of the apple in your mouth, to fully taste it. When we are mindful, we are immersed in the moment and living it fully.

Mindfulness is an excellent tool for overcoming both stress and anxiety, as it guides awareness, and brings the mind into the present moment instead of being lost somewhere in the past or future. It is simple but not always easy: We have lived our lives being caught up in ruminating about the past, worrying about the future, or involved in cognition about the present, so it takes effort, attention and awareness to be in the present moment. That being said, researches have found that the happiest people are the ones who are able to be present; the people who are mindful.

Free Resource: *For more information around mindfulness, including articles, podcasts, and recorded mindful meditations, check out Dr. Ron Siegel's (author of many books including 'The Mindfulness Solution' and 'The Extraordinary Gift of Being Ordinary') website at www.drronsiegel.com*

Meditating

Meditation is one of the best ways to practice mindfulness, and has been found to be incredibly supportive in reducing anxiety in individuals. In fact, the overall health and wellness benefits of meditation are almost exclusively second to none.

On a personal note, mindful meditation truly changed my life. As an anxious, stressed-out, workaholic, Type A personality with the assorted health impacts that one would expect to accompany that lifestyle including an ulcer by my early twenties, I finally found peace when I found meditation. In fact, it was so impactful for me, and the changes to my health and wellbeing were so significant that several years ago I left a 25-

year career in corporate life in order to teach mediation and mindfulness as a full time Health and Wellness Educator.

Among countless other benefits, meditation has been found to:

- Reduce stress, anxiety and depression
- Reduce blood pressure
- Reduce "bad" cholesterol levels
- Reduce chronic pain
- Reduce ruminative thought patterns
- Reduce inflammation
- Reduce gastrointestinal issues
- Reduce the size of the amygdala
- Increase one's levels of compassion and sense of wellbeing
- Increase cognitive abilities including memory
- Support immune system functioning
- Improve sleep
- Improve nutrient absorption

I could go on (and on, and on, and on…) about the benefits of meditation, however, a simple google search of "Why is meditation good for you" will do the trick.

"Mindfulness meditation doesn't change life.
Life remains as fragile and unpredictable as ever.
Meditation changes the heart's capacity to accept life as
it is. It teaches the heart to be more accommodating,

not by beating it into submission, but by making it clear that accommodation is a gratifying choice."

– Sylvia Boorstein

Mindful Practice: Breath Meditation

- Sit in a comfortable position with your eyes closed or softly gazing

- Allow your body to feel heavy and supported, gravity gently pulling your shoulders down from your neck

- Become aware of the fact that you are inside of a body that is breathing

- Allow your body to breathe normally; there is nothing for you to do, nowhere for you to be, and nothing for you to control

- Connect with the internal and external physical sensations that are occurring in your torso; you may notice that you feel your chest and shoulders rising and falling with the inhalation and exhalation, your belly gently and softly moving in and out, or the sensation of your lungs expanding and contracting as you breathe…

- Allow for yourself to become immersed in the sensations of breathing

- If you find that your mind begins to wander, that is normal. Gently, lovingly and non-judgementally simply bring your awareness back to the sensations of the breath in your body

That's it! That's meditation. There are so many different meditations to choose from in order to find the one(s) that resonate(s) best for you. Like every other practice in the guide, it's about giving different things a try and seeing what works.

Resonating

In the words of neuroscientist and author of the book *Your Resonant Self*, Sarah Peyton describes resonance as "the true experience two humans have where one has a warm inquiry about the other and the other says, "Yes, you understand me." When we resonate with someone, it provides immediate relief to our nervous system and simultaneously reduces levels of anxiety and stress. As humans, we are hard-wired to seek connection (another example of why mirror neurons are so pivotal) so when we become connected, we experience a feeling of safety. This is where, once again, the benefits of having a trusted person to speak with – a family member, a friend, a therapist – can be such an invaluable addition to our health and wellness. However, one of the many benefits of being an evolved mammal, is that we possess the cognitive ability to offer resonance to ourselves. We can utilize self-compassion to ask ourselves (with softness and warmth), "Hey, (insert your name here) …what's the matter, what are you feeling?" and when an authentic response arises, we can then access our creative and communicative minds to say, "Yes, of course that feeling makes sense. It comes from somewhere and that matters. You're okay." In essence, we can connect with *ourselves* in order to move back into regulation.

> **Mindful Reminder:** *View stress and anxiety for what they are - a state of defence or physiological distress…they are saying to you, "My physiology is disrupted – do something!" Ask yourself, "What can I offer you in this moment to help you to know that you are safe?" – It may be something as simple as a trip to the washroom, something to eat, or a different train of thought. If your anxiety is signalling something more than what just a "quick fix" can address, then make a date to be with yourself later to figure out what needs to change – and keep the date*

Injecting Some Humor

A few weeks ago, a day after a long road trip, I woke up with an unusual and uncharacteristic intense pain in my left calf.

I turned to my husband and announced, "It's leg cancer." Keith faced me with a bewildered look and said, "Why do you always have to go to the worst possible place?", to which I flatly replied, "Fine. It's a blood clot." Although that really *is* where my mind first goes (as I'm sure that many of you reading this book can understand), he and I both laughed.

Being able to have a sense of humor around life, including situations and ourselves, can act as a wonderful buffer to different emotions such as stress, anxiety and anger. The joke is that Keith and I both *know* that I go there, so why not poke a little fun at how silly our minds can be sometimes?

Often, we humans can look back at something that had been difficult for us at the time, and laugh about the situation or our reaction to it. Knowing that, is it at all possible for us to see that maybe we can find the humor in life sooner rather than later and save ourselves some of the grief and pain of being so upset in the moment? Although this may not be an appropriate modality *all of the time*, it may be something that you find useful in befriending your stress or anxiety even *some* of the time, and any improvement is still an improvement.

Laughing

Have you ever laughed when it was really inappropriate (such as in the middle of an argument, during grace at a family gathering, or at a funeral) or known of someone else who has? There is actually a reason for that: Laughing is a natural way of dispelling activation energy that is present in the body. Many people can't help themselves from laughing in situations that are not funny. It's not about 'funny' at that point, the body is taking control of the ship and releasing energy in a quick and efficient way; just as some people sigh unconsciously to reduce tension and anxiety, some people do it through laughing.

A few years ago, while on a WestJet flight home, the flight attendant made an announcement: "Ladies and gentlemen, as we begin our descent, I would like to bring to your attention to the fact that we have someone on board today celebrating their 100th birthday!" Many of the passengers on the plane, myself included, burst into applause. When the clapping died down, the flight attendant continued, "So as you depart the plane today, please wish the captain a 'Happy Birthday'!" We all laughed, as the joke did exactly what it was meant to do: reduce anxiety for what might be an anxious time.

If your body instinctively knows that laughing is good for you, then consider doing it more often purposely. Is there a comedy that you enjoy? Are there movies that make you laugh like a hyena? (Some of our favorites include "Just Go with It" starring Adam Sandler and Jennifer Aniston and "Fifty First Dates" with Adam Sandler and Drew Barrymore. Another movie with funny parts is "Grown Ups." Keith is a huge Seinfeld fan, and often bursts into fits of laughter even *recalling* one of his favorite scenes for me, whereas others in my life still swear by Monty Python movies or Mr. Bean.)

Perhaps you can find a joke that works for you:

A woman in an interview is asked by the interviewer, "What would you consider to be your worst trait?" The woman thinks about it for a moment and says, "Honesty." The interviewer says, "Well, I hardly think that honesty is a bad trait!" to which the woman replies, "I don't care what the hell you think!"

Just as slow exhalations and yawning signify to our brain that we are safe, so too, does laughing.

Giving Your Body What It Needs

I was fascinated and thrilled to hear about something called "Push Therapy" being used in the treatment of individuals who have experienced the trauma of being unable to 'fight back' at some point in their lives. This intervention involves working with a trauma specialized therapist who supports the individual in pushing hard against an object. This action has been found in some cases to help in releasing activated energy that was unable to be expressed at the time of a prior event. Basically, what the body didn't get to do in the past, it gets to do now.

Connect with your body and just see what it wants from you. Often, simply warmly inquiring to oneself in a moment of reflection will help you to hear what your intuition is asking for. There have been times in my past, especially as an adolescent, when my body was screaming for me to run, so I did. In fact, many times in my teens while living in a household that was especially dysfunctional, I would run as far, and as fast, and for as long as I could and then when I couldn't run another step, I would slowly walk back. As an adult, there have been times that merely imagining that I was running around the world was enough to satisfy my activation of flight (due to wanting to run away from work, or any other stressful activation). One of the youths that I work with told me that when he's really mad, he goes out into the woods where nobody can see him and he pounds his fists into the ground. It's not that he is imagining hitting anyone when he does it (I asked), it's just that he feels like hitting something and feels better when it's over. That is a perfect example of discharging pent up fight energy in a healthy way. What does your body need from you? What is it silently begging for? Maybe you need a hug, some time in solitude, a vacation, a night off from household duties, or the opportunity to scream into a pillow (also an example of discharging fight energy). There are two ways in particular that mammals will discharge pent up energy from a nervous system activation: One is to release tears. So, if you feel like what you need is a good cry, then give yourself the gift of a good cry.

> **Personal sharing:** *On more than one occasion during the creation of this book and wanting to make it as perfect for you as I could, I (ironically) experienced feelings of overwhelm and exhaustion. More than once, I found myself thinking, "I'm so tired – so lost as to where to go next - I just want to cry!" On one such occasion, I stopped typing, sat back, and said silently and lovingly to myself, "Okay Honey, you go ahead and cry then; you get all of your cries out. I'm right here to be with you and we'll do this*

together." My body softened immediately but no cries came; my body just needed to know that it had been heard and acknowledged with compassion. Simply the witnessing of myself, the personal attunement, was all I needed in order to move my system back into regulation

Mindful Tip: *The pre-frontal cortex acts as 'the adult in the room' and comparatively, the amygdala acts as 'the child in the room'. When you become aware of the fact that the 'child' is in charge, take control back with a thought such as, "As the functional adult in the room, how can I best support the part of me that feels incapable right now?"*

The second automatic stress-reducing action is to shake. In fact, in a study done with military personnel, it was discovered that soldiers who self-reported as having thwarted the body's response to shake after a stressful event (through tucking their hands into their underarms or holding their body parts down) were significantly more likely to suffer from Post-Traumatic Stress Disorder (PTSD). You may be or know someone who unconsciously (or habitually) shakes their leg or foot, or constantly stums their fingers as yet another form of bodily genius to self-regulate. I found it fascinating, albeit not surprising, that new research indicates that individuals who suffer with Restless Leg Syndrome tend to have a past-history of not being able to 'run' (express flight activation). Hence, what the body was not able to do in the past, it is now trying to express. Our illnesses are not our enemy, they are often a loving friend that is trying to communicate with us. Overall health and wellbeing increase dramatically when we listen to our bodies before they need to yell. If it feels like you might have some excess activation and it would be a match for you, you may want to consider engaging in some ecstatic dancing complete with hand and leg shakes or a personal version of the Hokey Pokey. If it feels right, you may want to make some noise while you do it. (I am absolutely not kidding; try it out and check in with yourself to see if there is any sense of relief.)

Continuing with honoring your body and providing yourself with what you need, perhaps it is time to face the fact that your intuition is begging for you to find a new job, to make sense of feeling torn between two authorities, or to exit a relationship that is toxic for you. As I offer in the book *Finding Yourself Again: Making Your Way Back to You*, just because you identify what your body means doesn't mean that you need to take immediate action; there are times when that is an appropriate action, and there are times when it is prudent to simply decipher next steps. Just asking yourself what you really, *really* need is a good start.

Mindful Reflection: Connecting with Oneself

It can be very easy and tempting for us to point the finger at other people in our lives and express to them what they are not providing for us. If you become aware of the fact that you blame others for what you are not receiving, connect with yourself:

- If you are wanting to be soothed in a better way from someone else, *reflect*: Do I already soothe myself? How good am I at soothing myself? In which ways could I improve?

- If you are looking for another person to spend more time with you, *reflect*: Do *I* spend enough time with me? How good am I at spending time with myself? How could I do a better job of spending time with myself?

- If you are upset with the way that someone speaks with you, *reflect*: How do I speak to myself? How good am I with my self-talk? In which ways could I improve my self-talk?

This reflection is by no means intended to be a free pass for someone in your life who is not providing you with what you need or treating you respectfully. However, many of us, myself included, can at times be guilty of projection – placing blame on others for something that we are not willing to face in ourselves. Interestingly, as we become better at our own self-care and self-treatment, the expectations of the treatment we receive from others begins soften and change because our needs are, to a large extent, already being met. Also, many of us can at times be guilty of treating others as they treat themselves and not as they deserve to be treated. When you embody self-respect and self-love, others will often quite naturally follow your lead.

Imagining *Not* Feeling Stressed

Although it seems as though some people are born to be anxious (a 3D image of our daughter in utero showed her already sucking her thumb), most of us get there through repeated practice. Hence, feeling stressed becomes a habit, and as messed up as it seems, it can actually feel uncomfortably unfamiliar to be free of negative emotions. Just like getting rid of any bad habit, such as smoking or drinking too much, we may need to replace a bad habit with a good one. This begins first by asking yourself, "Who would I be without that stressful thought? Who would I be if I was no longer anxious? What would my life look like if I no longer suffered from anxiety? How would I feel? How would I speak? What would I *do*?"

Mindful Tip: *The reason that children are able to let go of their emotions isn't because they have a technique to do so, it is because they haven't yet learned how to hold onto them. If learning how to let go of your anxiety does not work for you, is it possible for you to imagine unlearning holding on to it in the first place?*

Coregulating

Humans are mammals and mammals are designed to crave the comfort of other mammals. A baby needs to learn how to regulate, which is why being comforted, held, loved and attuned to (most especially when upset) as an infant is so important. However, even well-adjusted, normally-regulated adults need help sometimes when the nervous system has been activated and we just can't get ourselves back. Being in the presence of another human being that is properly regulated is easily sensed by our mirror neurons and by our own nervous system, and works to reduce all types of difficult emotional states including stress, anxiety, depression and anger. (Hence, "Wow, just being *near* that person makes me feel better for some reason…") It isn't about being an emotional vampire or overly-dependant on another (it is important to seek help if this is a personal default, as it indicates a need to establish a deeper wellspring of self-regulation and resilience techniques), but about temporarily 'borrowing' the nervous system of another when yours is not functioning at full capacity in the moment – much akin to 'getting a jump start' from another motor when your car battery isn't working properly. There are many times when reducing stress or anxiety isn't about being "fixed," it's about being attuned to. If human interaction is limited, or not available, then close proximity to another regulated mammal, such as a mammalian pet, will also help to reduce stress and anxiety levels.

Mindful Exercise: Orienting

If you are alone while you are experiencing stress or anxiety, you may find it benefit to orient yourself:

- If it is safe to do so, sit down or ensure that you are supported as you stand (supported by the ground, or supported by the wall or a table)

- Take a long, comfortable, slow, deep breath

- Move your head very slowly from one side of the room to the other as you take in your surroundings; what color are the walls? What texture is the flooring? What objects in the room grab your attention?

- Notice that nobody else is in the room with you

- Become aware of the fact that if you are safe, and that if nobody is in the room with you, then the stress or anxiety is internal; you are actually okay in this moment

The act of taking a deep breath, moving your head very slowly from side to side (like a lion surveying the Serengeti, knowing that there are no predators around) and engaging in external sensing as well as 'naming' what you see, all work to activate and engage the ventral vagal branch of the parasympathetic nervous system and bring you back into a state of regulated balance.

Involving Water

Many people find the properties of water to be cleansing and restorative. If this is something that you resonate with, you may choose to indulge in a bath or shower, to go for a swim, to head to the nearest lake, ocean or stream, or to listen to recorded sounds of a babbling brook or the rain falling. For some people, even looking at a picture of water can be nourishing for their sense of wellbeing.

Dodging the Hook

Although it's not always the case, the people who know us the best tend to be the people in our lives that know just what to bait the hook with in order to catch us; that includes ourselves and our own 'hooking' thoughts. Become mindful of the 'hooks' that people, events, emotions, thoughts, and triggers create in your life. If your overbearing in-law makes a comment about your culinary skills, recognize, "Oh, there it is – there's the hook. I am going to ignore it." If a colleague comes in to work in yet another bad mood and says something snappy to you, consider thinking, "I'm not going to get hooked. I don't have to even interpret this; this does not belong to me." And if you find that you are in a situation where there are simply too many hooks in the water for you to avoid, consider utilizing some self-care by swimming to another location.

Mindful Tip: *It is easy for us to become "hooked" by wondering what someone else is thinking, or getting caught up in anxiety or stress by thinking that perhaps we have upset them. The truth is this: If a person is upset with us or has something to say, they will let us know, and if not, it may be time to reassess the relationship*

Going with the Flow

Sticking with the water theme:

- See if it's possible for you to not take life so seriously and just allow yourself to go with the flow

- Let the trials and tribulations of life be like water off a duck's back

- Recognize that thoughts, emotions, and events in life all come and go like waves; bills come and go, anxiety comes and goes, many relationships come and go, money comes and goes but the ocean still remains

- Rainy days bring new growth

- Remain grounded yet flexible, like seaweed (that one is my favorite, and I use it all the time as a visualization technique)

Savouring

To savour something is to relish, appreciate and delight in it. The acts of savouring and delighting are only available to us during moments of safety. The more moments of safety that we have, the more that we accumulate, and the more that we accumulate, the more that we have. Life is not about punishment; it is about enjoying…savouring…the ride. Look for things that you appreciate, enjoy, or delight in every day and then savour them…relish in them for as long as you can, even if it is just a few seconds. Consider starting each morning by placing the numbers 1-3 or 1-5 or 1-10 on a page, and then look for and notice things to savour. After savouring something, write it down and then keep looking; we build our resources one step, one micro-moment at a time. Here are just a few suggestions for things that you may find you can savour:

- The feeling of being in a warm bed
- Comfortable pajamas
- The sensation of a warm cup of tea, coffee or hot chocolate in your hands
- Eating something
- A satiated stomach after something to eat
- Sharing a smile with someone
- The sound of laughter between two strangers

- The fact that you can press a button and the tv turns on
- Looking into someone's eyes and noticing the different flecks of color
- Having the sense of hearing or touch or taste or sight or smell
- The knowledge that someone cares about you (and even if this is difficult for you to believe, I promise you that even strangers such as myself, many strangers, care about you deeply; please consider savouring that)

Mindful Tip: *The voices of stress and anxiety try to convince us that the way out of stress and anxiousness is to hold tighter and to push harder. The truth is that the way out of stress and anxiousness is to loosen the grip and to stop forcing. When you let go of the fight, you may realize that in all actuality, there was no fight to be had*

Reframing Activation

So often, stress and anxiety are rarely about what is actually happening in the moment and more often about our *perception* of what is actually happening in the moment. Anxiousness and stress are simply forms of energy, and we can consciously choose to adjust our perception in order to work *with* the energy instead of fight *against* it.

<u>Mindful Tip:</u> *Imagine stress as a horse; instead of running from it, move towards it, calling, "Whoa, easy, easy…" and strap a saddle on its back so that you can harness its power*

Activation of our sympathetic nervous system is not always a bad thing. While it is true that anxiety mobilizes our fight or flight response, so does competing in a race or working under the pressure of a tight deadline. There are times in life when healthy activation is not only helpful, but necessary in the completion of everyday tasks. Therefore, instead of perpetuating stress or anxiousness through habitual thought-loops, we can interrupt the stress response by reframing our perception of what is happening.

If you notice that you are stressed or anxious because of something that needs to be done, try reframing the situation with something like, "Oh, Anxiety! I'm so glad you're here! I can really use all of the energy that you're providing me with in order to complete the task ahead of me!" It has been stated that, "anxiety is enthusiasm without the breath." Knowing that; <u>breathe</u>. "Whew! Okay, Stress – let me just get a hold of my breathing so that I can think clearly and rationally about how best to utilize all of the resources that you're giving me access to." Stress and anxiety are merely activated energy that can be utilized and maximized in order to support us in feeling ready, alert, energized, quick-thinking and hyper-tuned to senses.

Merely the decision alone to focus on the breath is half the battle:

Mindful Practice: 4 x 4 x 4 Breathing

- Softly, slowly and deeply breathe in while gently and silently counting to 4 – "one…two…three…four…"

- Softly, slowly, and deeply breathe out while gently and silently counting down from four – "four…three…two…one…"

- Repeat 4 times or until you feel that you have activated your parasympathetic nervous system

Mindful Tip: *Anytime you remember, take a moment to notice anything that's different after you have been successful in settling your nervous system. As you become more practiced at activities that support regulation, you may be able to recognize the emotions and sensations that accompany parasympathetic activation. Generally, this may include a naturally slower breath, softening of muscles, a general feeling of relaxation, and access to calm and rational thinking that may not have been accessible to you a moment ago*

Activation of the stress response can be akin to the cacophony that accompanies the various musicians who are warming up until they receive some sort of direction. Getting a hold of your physiology puts you squarely and directly in the position of being the orchestrator of your orchestra.

Accepting Things and People as They Are

<u>Mindful Reflection:</u> *Reflect for a moment on how this phrase lands for you:*

"If I am trying to change another person or the outside world, I will be waiting for a very long time."

Refusing to accept a person or a situation is almost certainly a recipe for creating anxiety. It is easy and tempting to get caught up in thoughts such as, "But if things were different, then I would be happy," or "If they would just change the way I want them to, everything would be better." These statements remind me of one of my most favorite definitions of stress: "When things in life don't go the way we want(ed) them to." Try as I might, I still can't say for sure that I know what the point of life is, but I can say for certain that it isn't to get things in life to go the way we want(ed) them to.

Frankly put, to choose acceptance is to make the choice to release stress and anxiety. At the very least, it is making the choice to loosen their grips on us.

Mindful Practice: I Accept This

- Sit or stand comfortably and slowly survey your surroundings

- Find something small, possibly even insignificant about your surroundings that mildly displeases you. Perhaps it is a picture that is hanging crookedly, a stain on the floor, a dent in the wall, a pile of clutter, something that needs to be cleaned, or a to-do list that is taunting you

- Accept that this particular thing is this way for this moment. It doesn't mean that it doesn't need to be changed or corrected, or that you don't wish that it was different, it simply means that in this moment, it is how or what it is

- Say either silently or aloud, "I accept this."

- **Breathe. Relax. Release.** Let go of your resistance. This is how this thing is in this moment whether you like it or not and fighting it simply creates an unhealthy activation in your body

- Repeat again, either silently or out loud, "I accept this."

- Breathe deeply

- Relax your muscles

- Release your need for this thing to be different from what it is, because in this moment, it is not different from what it is; it is what it is, whether you like or accept it or not

- I accept this

- Investigate what it feels like in your body and in your mind to just release (or at the very least, pause) your resistance to this fact of reality

Mindful Tip: *The more that you practice acceptance of the "small stuff" in life, the easier it gets to accept some of the "big stuff" in life*

For a deeper practice, if it is comfortable for you (feel free to disengage in this practice – any practice – if it becomes overwhelming or uncomfortable for you), try this one:

- Sit or stand where you are comfortably supported

- Allow your eyes to close or gently place a soft gaze on something that will not distract you

- Bring to mind something in your life that is difficult for you to accept (a person, an event, etc.)

- Acknowledge that this thing, event or person already exists as it is; that is undeniable. The person is who they are, the event has already happened, etc. This is reality for this moment whether we like it or not, agree with it or not, or want it to change

- Silently or aloud, "I accept this."

- If you notice resistance, feel free to assure yourself however you need to. That may look something like, "I don't like this. I think it is _____ (wrong, bad, etc.), and I want it to change (or wish that it didn't happen, etc.), but I accept it.

- I accept that in this moment, this is true

- Breathe. Slowly and calmly, remain centered

- Relax. Relax your body. Relax into this statement

- Release. Let go of carrying this resistance, even for just a moment; for this one moment, accept that this is true and release the burden (even for a second) of fighting against it

- I accept this

- Investigate what it feels like in your body and in your mind to just release (or at the very least, pause) your resistance to this fact of reality

<u>Mindful Tip:</u> *When someone is struggling with stress or anxiety, two of the most helpful, compassionate, and supportive things that we can offer them are a regulated nervous system (remaining calm and grounded, while not being condescending about it) and gently inquiring to ourselves with kind curiosity and an open heart, "I wonder what this person's nervous system (or behavior) is trying to communicate to me right now?"*

There are many things that we can accept in the moment and then set an intention to change in the future (such as accepting the reality of Climate Change, but still making or lobbying for changes), however, you may find that after practicing this exercise it actually feels quite nice sometimes to make the decision to let go of burdens or baggage that doesn't necessarily belong to you. You may recognize that there is stuff that you have been carrying around that you didn't need to; that you spent (or are spending) your energetic resources on something that didn't get you anywhere. It is possible that with some baggage that you've been carrying with you, you may make the liberating and empowering choice to *not* pick it up again. If you have been in the habit of carrying the responsibilities of others, this doesn't mean that you no longer help others to get their backpacks on, it simply means that you make the decision to no longer carry someone else's backpack yourself.

> **<u>Mindful Tip:</u>** *Many of us put undue stress and anxiety into our lives by trying to get other people to change. When I find myself getting frustrated because I want my children or spouse to be a certain way "for their own good," I remind myself that people become who they were meant to be and that they are on a path that I cannot view from my own: The most loving and compassionate thing we can do for another is to accept them for who they are. There is no amount of effort that we could give that could teach a cat to bark*

Lastly, sometimes acceptance also includes 'taking the blow' for something we've done. Recognizing and acknowledging when we have erred so that we can rectify the situation promotes inner growth. Denial or hiding of mistakes or refusing to take ownership of what rightfully belongs to us (no judgement here, we've all been there) can be extremely an anxiety-provoking and stressful weight to carry. Although it takes strength, effort and courage to do it, character is built through changing ourselves in order to become who we want to be. Personally, through much (*much*) practice (just ask my family), I have become very good at authentically saying, "I am really sorry. That was wrong (or disrespectful, or thoughtless, or inconsiderate, or unnecessary, or mean…) of me and I shouldn't have done it. It won't happen again." Not only does this action reduce personal stress and anxiety levels, but more importantly, it also works to repair ruptures (which are a healthy and normal part of any relationship).

Staying with the Facts

When we purposely and consciously "stick to the facts," we can shift our focus from emotionality (the amygdala or "up" position) to cognition (the PFC or "balanced center"). This may look something like this: anxious or stressful thoughts about a traffic jam lead us to thoughts about being late for work, which then leads us to imagining being yelled at by our boss, which would then lead to thoughts of getting fired. After being fired, we would lose our home, and then of course that leads to thoughts of getting a divorce because of all the stress on the family… and the rest of the catastrophizing that so many of us are so good at. Staying with the facts looks like this: "I am sitting in the car. My hands are on the wheel. My car is on a road. There is a blue car behind me and a red car in front of me. My car is black. The temperature in my car is comfortable."

> **Gentle Reminder:** *Often, the goal is simply to interrupt unhealthful or negative habituated thought patterns and then to consciously choose a new pathway for our thoughts to learn. Just as anxiety has become a habit, we can train ourselves into a habit of relaxation and ease: The 'muscles' we continually utilize get stronger*

Spending Time in Nature

"Everything that slows us down and forces patience, everything that sets us back into the slow circles of nature, is a help. Gardening is an instrument of grace."

– May Sarton

An immediate way to decrease levels of stress and anxiety is to spend time in nature. The benefits of getting outside are as deep as the ocean and as vast as the sky:

- Sunshine often accompanies being outdoors and we all know that with sunshine comes a healthy dose of vitamin D. Vitamin D is linked to lowered blood pressure, improved brain functioning, improved sleep and it has been found to reduce stress, anxiety, depression, and seasonal affective disorder
- The fresh air in nature cleans our lungs, increases energy levels, strengthens immune functioning, improves mood and has been found to improve digestion
- Nature itself is full of healing and health-promoting benefits, such as reducing stress hormones, which reflects with helping us to have less fear, stress and anger. Not only does it reduce our stress hormones, but it increases hormones that help us to feel positive

emotions, such as joy and gratitude. It has even been found to reduce pain levels. In fact, even looking at photos of nature has been found to produce these qualities in humans.

<u>**Free Resource:**</u> *For a quick mood enhancer that includes beautiful pictures of nature, check out the six-minute film on You Tube entitled, "Gratitude: The Short Film by Louie Schwartzberg."*

- When we go outside, we tend to get exercise while we're out there, whether we're walking, running, hiking, swimming, biking or playing. The benefits of exercise are also countless, which means that nature just keeps giving and giving
- Simply laying on the lawn, working in a garden, walking barefoot on the beach, or watching the clouds as they dance or laze in the sky all work to reduce stress and anxiety

If you can't get out, that's okay too! Bring some flowers into your home from outside or buy a plant. Open your window, or post up some pictures of your favorite nature scenes. Stand out on your balcony if you have one.

And if none of these things are available to you, even just *thinking* about nature; imagining its beauty and brilliance, still provides you with health benefits, including lowered levels of cortisol.

Using Your Imagination for Good

It is easy for anyone to get caught up in ruminative or stressful thinking, including over-planning, over-analyzing or over-worrying. When you catch that your mind has wandered away and is producing activation in your body, choose to move your thoughts to a more helpful location. Instead of using those amazing planning skills or that creative imagination to think about what could go wrong, or what should have gone better, shift those same cognitive abilities to focus on what could go right or what has gone well in the past (if you choose not to stay in the present moment). While it is true that we can think of all of the terrible things that might happen in the future, it is also true that we could train our brain to start thinking about all of the amazingly wonderful things that might happen in the future. You can choose to allow your mind and thought processes to lead you down the path of a fiery pit, or you can consciously select thoughts that will lead your mind and thought processes to an open and beautiful meadow. One path leads to illness and the other to health; choose to have your imagination work *for* you and not *against* you.

Naming the Persona

Dr. Richard Schwartz reports that he developed Internal Family Systems (IFS) Therapy in response to many of his clients sharing with him that they felt as though they had different "parts" of themselves. It is common to feel as though there are parts of us that are bossy or mean, parts of us that are scared and parts of us that are loving. When we become aware of these parts using different methods for metacognition (meta meaning "above" and cognition meaning "thinking"; basically a term that is used for when we become aware of the fact that we are thinking, which means that there is something more…such as a soul…behind the actual thoughts that are being thought), it invites and allows for us to have a different experience of our inner world and to not get so caught up in thinking that just because we think something that it is true. When we can name the persona(s) inside of us, we can provide ourselves with space to question our own thoughts. For example, one might imagine that their anxiety is an older mother-in-law type persona named Worrying Wendy that runs around wringing her hands over everything. Anytime you notice that you are engaging in anxious thoughts, you may say to something to yourself such as, "There's Worrying Wendy again, all upset and trying to convince me that I'll never get everything done on time. Thanks Wendy, but I'm working hard and it will all get finished." This type of naming (different from 'Name It to Tame It' where one names the emotions and physiological sensations) creates some room for humor or entertainment with our thoughts. "Hey, Negative Neil – if all you're going to do is tell me that this day sucks and that I suck and that my family sucks, I'm going to invite Positive Paul over to see what he has to say instead." Again, this is an opportunity to stop a habituated thought process in its tracks in order to build new territory.

Mindful Tip: *Emotions are just emotions – they are not facts, they are not who you are, and with practice you can learn to let them go. Emotions are simply energy that we do not have to choose to follow*

Identifying Separation

If you find that you tend to become anxious or triggered by the emotions of another, mindfully become aware that you are separate from them. During an uncomfortable conversation, this may look something like silently thinking to yourself: "I recognize that I am here and you are there. I am standing here. I can feel my feet on the ground. I can feel my hands attached to my arms. That is you over there, and this is me right here. We are separate. You are speaking and I am nodding. Now I am speaking and you are nodding. I am okay. I am separate." You may also find it helpful to do some investigative math, such as silently acknowledging, "Ten percent of this activation is mine. Ninety percent of this activation is yours. I can calm down my activation level with relaxed breathing. I am okay."

Mindful Reflection: Are you, or do you know a fawner?

__ Consistently taking care of people or situations

__ Getting praised for how 'together' you are, how generous you are, how well you take care of others or have everything 'under control'

__ Appear to be fine on the outside, but are struggling on the inside – trouble sleeping, feeling exhausted all of the time, rapid heartbeat

*If so, this is good to recognize! Fawning is one of the lesser-known "F's" of activation. It has evolved as part of our mammalian traits. More typically found in females, it was less detected as a stress response, because many pioneering tests were performed on males (who tend to be more prone to fight or flight responses). Be mindful of your fawning tendencies and when you notice that you are fawning; pause. Ask yourself, "*What does my nervous system need from me in this moment in order to feel safe and supported?*"

Having Faith

Anxiety and stress both have roots that stem from a lack of trust; in ourselves, others, the situation, or even life itself. The saying, "Let go and let God" has more than just deep religious roots; it also has incredibly significant biological merit. Leading neuroscientist and author of many books, including *How God Changes Your Brain*, Dr. Andrew Newberg asserts that having a positively-based faith system is one of the healthiest things that we can do for our brains. Indeed, believing in something that is bigger and more powerful than us allows us to let go of feeling the burden to have to carry the weight of the world on our shoulders. Whether the faith-system is religious or not does not matter; it just needs to be a hopeful and trusting belief in something other than yourself. You may choose to believe in a God or gods, in the Universe, or an omnipotent benevolent Source. Perhaps you have faith in karma, or in your family heritage. Maybe it is faith in yourself. You could choose to have faith in humankind; we are all connected. The biology of mirror neurons is a perfect example – these cells that fire whether we are performing and action or witnessing the action of another truly indicate that what others do (even if they are strangers) affects us, and that what we do to others, we do to ourselves: That's a pretty amazing and truly miraculous thing. The importance here is that you have a positive belief system that allows you to trust in life; to let go of having to know everything, of having to fix everything and of having to do everything. Wouldn't it be nice to simply trust that there is a plan? Let go and have faith.

> **Free Resource:** *Many people have found space from their stress or anxiety through some of the principals used in The Diamond Approach. You can check out if this may be a match for you at www.diamondapproach.org*

It is when we are feeling stressed or anxious that we most desperately seek an orientation of calm, however, we need to empower ourselves by finding it. There is effort required in moving from who we are to who we want to be. Thankfully, the list of neuro-calming and nervous system regulating choices available to us is forever endless. Along with all the other myriad offers that you have already read, here are a few more:

1. Pause. Slow down if you are rushing
2. Walk around in your bare feet in order to feel more grounded
3. Look around your environment slowly, accessing and utilizing the amazing tracking ability of your eyes
4. Swing in a hammock
5. Utilize aromatherapy
6. Speak with someone you trust that cares about your wellbeing
7. Put a hand on your forehead or one hand on your forehead and the other behind your head
8. Give yourself a hug
9. Use your favorite paramedical modality, such as a visit to your acupuncturist or massage therapist
10. Dance
11. Connect with anywhere at all in your body that feels soft, neutral, relaxed or painless. If so, direct your attention to that one spot (even if it is the pinky toe on your right foot)
12. Reflect on the things that you used to do for fun before you were stressed or anxious and go and do one of those activities
13. Place a hand or hands over your heart

14. Pay attention to a material object and allow yourself to become immersed in investigating it
15. Listen to, and identify different bird calls
16. Feel something in your hands, exploring the way it feels
17. Use visualization, such as imagining yourself being in a location that is soothing for you, or that you are as unshakable as a mountain, as flexible as seaweed or as rooted as a magnificent oak tree. If you're finding yourself too challenged in a situation to do anything else, try just imagining that you are a grey rock: emotionless and solid, but still okay. Breathe
18. Remember that you will not always feel activated or stuck; this too shall pass
19. Make love with yourself or your partner
20. Ground to feeling supported by another person (reflect upon a moment in your life when you have felt supported by another and become immersed in the sensations that the feeling created for you)
21. Spend time gardening
22. Write
23. Knit (lots of younger people are finding the benefits of this extraordinarily helpful 'pastime')
24. Read a good book
25. Watch the clouds
26. Draw, sketch or doodle

27. Recognize that things are constantly fluid and moving, see if you can notice even the slightest of shifts as you breathe deeply; curiously investigate if you are able to go to that place. If so, can you expand that feeling?

Mindful Tip: *Other activities that promote mental, emotional and physical balance are those that involve movements of left to right, such as boxing, running or drumming, swimming, playing the piano or even just crawling around on the floor*

Just like all the other techniques in this book, nobody needs to know what you do in order to self-soothe and self-regulate. For example, as a grown woman, mother, and professional, I used to bring a Sesame Street coloring book with me every time we went camping. Time melted away as I pressed as hard or as softly as I wanted to while coloring Big Bird or Ernie. If it works, who cares? I also love finding shapes and patterns in stucco or textured tiles – sometimes I see clowns or foxes or anteaters; I allow my imagination to just run wild. Often, the expressions on the faces of the animals that I 'see' offer an excellent representation of my own conscious or unconscious mood (happy, sad, frightened, angry…). If doing something that you like, likes you (is good for your nervous system), then that's what matters! Life isn't meant to be so serious all the time; allow yourself to be silly sometimes and to lighten up.

Lastly, I wanted to share with you a story of using visualization as a support system to help the body 'remember' how to feel calm:

After our car accident, Liz (very young at the time) started getting eczema, which is something that had never happened before. It was so bad, covering her entire body, that we had to take her to a top specialist because all of the other multiple doctors we visited could not give us a diagnosis; none of them had ever seen anything like it (the guesses included hand and mouth disease, severe chicken pox or a parvovirus infection, but the fact that she had it everywhere – including the bottom of her feet) ruled all of these guesses out. My heart broke as little Elizabeth noticed that people would stop to stare at her, or would move in order to get as far away from her as they could. The specialist diagnosed it as "one of the worst cases of eczema that she had ever seen", but eczema nonetheless. She prescribed cortisol (hydrocortisone) and told me to smear it all over Liz's tiny little body. After a test of one smear bleached her skin, I spoke with the psychologist I was seeing in Self Regulation Therapy to get her opinion. Although she doesn't treat children, she suggested that I help Liz to visualize her skin being healed in order to remind her skin of what it can do. That night as coached, as I laid with Liz for her nighttime snuggles, I invited her to create a magical cream in her mind, complete with color, texture, taste, smell, and even sound, and had her tell me how it would feel against her skin and how quickly her skin would heal after she 'put it on.' With a little bit of extra magic (including a secret animal that I have forever been sworn to secrecy about), she then pictured rubbing it on her skin and imagined her skin healing – she immersed herself in imagining her skin calm, smooth and painless. The very next morning after our first 'session' together, the spots had already begun drying up and no new spots were present. Within three days (20/30-minute process repeated each night with different 'potion creams'), all of her eczema had cleared and was in the healing stages. That was it. Done. We required our 'magic' a few more times for flare-ups, and the eczema would clear within a day or two. Aside from that one smear patch, we never used cortisol on her skin. Her nervous system benefited from a gentle reminder that she was safe enough to be able to settle back into regulation.

> *In no way am I advocating to disregard the advice of a doctor, nor am I suggesting that there are natural healing techniques for every medical situation, however what I *am* advocating is to consider getting a second opinion from an expert when something doesn't feel right to you; bringing the body back to homeostasis is a crucial foundation of health and, depending on the ailment, can sometimes be done through various measures *

Below are a few of the suggestions that many people are tired of hearing about (insert eyeroll), but with a twist: This will be short, and address some of the *why* behind the recommendations:

Getting Enough Sleep

Sleep is quite often the first thing to be compromised when we are feeling stressed or anxious, however, it should be just the opposite. The majority of adults need between 7-9 hours of sleep per 24-hour period in order to perform optimally (youth and adolescents require 8 -10). A dysregulated nervous system is what keeps us from sleeping, however, in yet another perpetuating cycle, when we do not get enough sleep, the amygdala senses a threat and mobilizes our fight or flight system, increasing levels of stress and anxiety. When we do more relaxing things throughout the day, we prime ourselves for better sleep. Even little things like coloring on your coffee break or meditating for a few minutes before starting your day can create significant improvements to sleep. (Ever notice that you tend to sleep better on vacation? One of the reasons has to do with the relaxing choices you make during the day…) Simply knowing that is it normal to become stressed or anxious in bed (your nervous system finally has some quiet time with which it can communicate with you) can be helpful. A very common comment in our house is, "Things *always* look worse at night. Let's pause and look at it again in the morning."

Free Resource: *Have trouble falling asleep? My son swears by 'The Military Method' taught to help military personnel fall asleep under any type of conditions:*

1. *Relax your entire face, including your forehead, eyes, and entire mouth*
2. *Drop your shoulders to release tension. You may want to do one side and then the other several times. Let your hand drop beside your body.*

3. *Let out long, slow exhalations, and allow for your chest and belly to relax*
4. *Relax all of the muscles in your legs*
5. *Clear your mind and picture only a relaxing scene. Imagine that you are lying comfortably on a beach, nestled in the warm sand with a cool breeze, or supported in a comfortable bed of grass while lazily watching the clouds move slowly in the sky, or lying safely on an inflatable mat in the middle of a peaceful and serene lake…*
6. *If you prefer, simply think the words, "don't think, don't think, don't think…" for ten seconds*

It is said that, with practice, people can fall asleep in as little as 10 – 120 seconds. There is tons of information about "The Military Method" online, including videos on YouTube. This is one of my favorites: https://www.youtube.com/watch?v=FWGuy4oOQgQ

Eating a Proper Diet

Gut microbiome (often shortened to simply, "gut biome") consists of trillions of bacteria and other microbes, and plays a huge part in digestion and immune system functioning. The foods and beverages that we consume affect our gut biome, and our gut biome affects our physical, emotional and mental states. Instead of "You are what you eat," the full saying needs to be, "You are *physically, mentally, and emotionally affected by* what you eat." Therefore, diet can play a large part in feelings of stress and/or anxiousness. What constitutes a "proper diet" is as unique as you are. Some people need more protein than others while others need more carbs; your body will provide you with clues (such as headaches, lethargy, vitamin deficiencies, mood swings, digestive messages, etc.) to let you know what it needs. When we skip meals or do not consume the fuel that our body needs, the brain picks that up and sounds the alarm, both as a throw-back to the feast-or-famine days of our ancestors, as well as a signal that the body is not getting the fuel it needs to run efficiently. Not eating a diet that is suitable for our body can activate the sympathetic nervous system and result in feelings of stress or anxiousness. Simply asking yourself, "What can I do to be more proactive in supporting my gut health?" is an excellent place to begin. Remember that everything is cumulative; even the smallest of steps make a difference!

Exercising

Anxiety is an emotion, and emotions are simply energy in motion; motion that needs to be expressed. Everyone has nervous system activation – every day, multiple times a day. Humans are built to withstand this. A car cutting in front of you in traffic causes the seesaw to go up into sympathetic response, and avoiding a crash along with a nice deep sigh moves the seesaw back into neutral. Different scenarios, different levels of activation and then transition back to a calm and dependable ventral vagal parasympathetic nervous system. Easy-peasy. However, that nervous energy of fight or flight doesn't often get to work its way out of our system; if you didn't run to safety (flee) to avoid the car crash, or punch the other driver out (fight) – both of which would not be appropriate – then that activated energy may still be inside of your body. Exercise is a fast, efficient, and healthy way to expel the normal, everyday activations of being human.

> **<u>Mindful Tip:</u>** *Stress balls that you can hold in your hand and squish can be used discretely, and are another way of releasing accumulated stress or anxiety from the body*

Hydrating

Just as everyone has different needs for food consumption, water consumption needs also vary. Your body will let you know what it needs through signs such as headaches or lack of urination if you are dehydrated. Often the first and easiest hint that your body will provide to you that it needs more water is through the sensation of thirst. If you are thirsty, honor your body and drink more water. When we are dehydrated, the amygdala activates to let us know that we are in danger, resulting in fight or flight activation, which may include – you guessed it – stress or anxiety.

Part VIII: More Hows

"…thoughts are secondary to bodily sensations, and as the body relaxes our thoughts shift from sensing the world is dangerous, to being safe."

- *Dr. Peter Levine*

If you're not finding the information too exhaustive, we will continue with even more techniques for supporting and calming your nervous system.

Mindful Practice: Wiring Expansion

Stress and anxiety both cause (and are caused by) constriction in the body. Consciously tensing the body and then consciously relaxing the body works to override autopilot and put you back in charge:

- Without forcing, and without pain or strain, but with some effort (basically, what I'm trying to say here is, "don't hurt yourself!") consciously tighten your bodily muscles from your face to your toes and hold for ten seconds

- Now soften and release all of your muscles from the top of your head to your feet

- Staying with muscles soft and in a relaxed position, curiously and compassionately investigate how it *feels* to be inside of a body that is completely comfortable. Take your time

- Repeat as desired

<u>Mindful Practice: Synchronizing the Body</u>

- Inhaling deeply, slowly raise your arms in unison to your breath

- Exhaling slowly, lower your arms at the same rate of your breathing, returning them to your sides

- Repeat as desired

<u>Mindful Practice: Voo Breathing</u>

- Take a nice, easy breath in, allowing the belly and chest to gently fill with air

- On the exhalation, slowly make the sound "voo", visualizing that it starts from the stomach and works its way entirely out of your body

- Repeat as desired

- When you are ready to complete this exercise, remain quiet for a moment as you slowly and softly investigate any internal sensations. Are you experiencing any thoughts or images? Are there any feelings present? Are there any sensations of tingling or vibration lingering in the body? Do you sense any coolness or warmth anywhere? Notice if any of these sensations begin to slowly spread within the body. If so, how does it *feel* to have these sensations in your body?

Mindful Practice: Shifting Physiology

- Sit or stand in a position that overly exaggerates how you are currently feeling (for example, if you are feeling exhausted, allow your body to hunch over or if you are feeling tense, tense up your whole body)

- Feel on the inside how it feels to place your body into this position on the outside

- Now gently move into a posture that exemplifies how you would *like* to be feeling right now

- Take a moment to internally sense how it feels to place your body into this position on the outside

- Repeat as desired
    a. The point with this exercise is not necessarily to then *feel* the emotions of the posture that you moved into, the point of this exercise is to calm the nervous system. If your second position was one of "alertness," the goal is not necessarily to feel alert (although you may notice that do feel closer to that state); the goal is to feel safer or more settled in your body than when you began the exercise

Mindful Practice: The Sensation of Strength

- Become aware of the fact that you are in a body

- Softly connect with the sensations in your back

- Softly connect with the sensations of your hips and sit bones

- Softly connect with the sensations of your feet

- Softly connect with the sensations of your hands

- Gently allow your hands to open and close

- Place all of your awareness into your hands as you very slowly continue to open and close them

- Curiously investigate what happens internally as you close your hands. Are you able to connect with a feeling of strength as you close them?

- Curiously investigate any internal sensations as you slowly allow your hands to open. Are you able to sense any feelings of openness or receptivity in the body?

    b. Again, never forcing; simply inquiring within; is it at all possible for you to allow your internal state to gently mirror the external sensations of strength and allowing?

Part IX: A Poem for How

A couple of months ago, near the end of the schoolyear, there was a poetry contest held at my daughter's high school. Witnessing these youth express their deepest thoughts and emotions was an amazing and beautiful experience.

One poem in particular deeply touched my heart. It was written by a friend of Liz's, and to watch and hear Kate share her poem was to be infused with awe, inspiration and hope. As I listened to her words and felt her authenticity, I thought to myself, "*This poem needs to be shared with every single person in the world!*"

I was surprised and saddened when Kate's poem, entitled "How to be a Star" was not announced as the winning one, and the thought of it not being shared as it should just didn't feel right. With her permission, I am sharing Kate V.'s poem with you here; it is so incredibly fitting and I hope that it touches and moves your heart as it does mine. If only we had all learned the lessons that Kate has to share when we were younger…

How to be a Star

1. Gaze down at the world below you,

From high above the clouds.

Look around at the beauty that drifts around you in awe.

Don't worry about falling and know that you are exactly where you are meant to be in the galaxy.

2. Shine bright.

Dazzle, flash, glow, shimmer, and sparkle.

Be who you are,

I promise, you will illuminate the entire night sky with all who do the same.

3. Stand with others.

Surround yourself with like minded people and those who inspire you.

Together, you stand strong.

Together, you form constellations that continue to fascinate everyone.

From day dreamers to the world's greatest geniuses.

4. Be patient.

It takes time for everyone to see that beautiful glow.

It may take ten thousand years for your light to meet the eyes of your secret admirers down on earth.

But when it does, trust me, it will be worth your burn.

5. Don't let those giant stars get you down.

Never be ashamed of being small.

Those fellows burn through so much fuel keeping up such a reputation,

They are destined to explode,

You are destined to radiate across the night sky.

6. Embrace your age.

One million years? That's nothing.

One billion? That's genuinely something.

Accept all that you are and that you are becoming.

Getting older only means that you sparkle brighter.

7. Be unique.

Don't blend in.

Step out of line and make a statement.

Everyone thinks stars should be white, like a diamond.

The most powerful stars show their true colours.

They are blue like vast, almighty oceans.

8. Dance.

Dance freely without a care across the night sky.

Spin, twirl, leap, tango, waltz, and float.

Express the joy that is overflowing inside of you.

9. Be grateful.

Be grateful for all those other stars that help you achieve glory.

Be grateful for the peace and harmony that surrounds you.

Remember, that you were born with the gift of freedom placed in your hands.

Never forget that life is not an entitlement, it is a divine privilege.

10. Know that you embody hope.

Every single star in existence plays an essential role in accomplishing a better tomorrow.

A better solar system,

A better galaxy,

And a better universe.

We are all made of molecules, and those molecules are made up of ancient star dust.

Without those stars that shone ever so brightly long ago, where would you and I be today?

- High School Senior, Kate V.

Part X: The Most Powerful How

"It is not the mountains we conquer, but ourselves."

– Sir Edmund Hillary

As promised at the beginning of this guide, the most powerful "how" for overcoming stress and anxiety would be unveiled to you.

The reason that it comes at the end, is because the rest of the guide was necessary. Your most powerful tool for overcoming stress or anxiety is twofold:

1) Education
2) Awareness

The knowledge that you have gleaned from the information in this guide covers everything you need to know to in order to build your own "Overcoming Stress and Anxiety Toolkit." Firstly, being kind and supportive with yourself through the use of self-compassion. As the old adage states, "You catch more flies with honey," so too is it true that you will get to where you want to get faster and with more ease when you are sweet with yourself versus sour. Humaning is hard; it can be scary, and confusing, and sad, and angering and overwhelming. And of course, it can be stress-producing and anxiety-provoking. At times it can be all of those things together and more. So, if being human is hard, then go softly on yourself. Offer yourself all of the things that you would wish to receive from a benevolent caregiver: love, compassion, patience, understanding, wisdom, unconditional acceptance, forgiveness, and humor. Offer yourself some lightness to what can sometimes feel like an extremely heavy journey.

You now know that feeling stressed or anxious is not only completely normal, but that it is evolutionarily and biologically hardwired into your being: there is nothing wrong with you. There has never been anything wrong with you. Take a long, slow, deep inhalation and an even longer, slower, deeper exhalation as you allow that knowledge to permeate through your DNA: You are okay.

And you learned that even though you come by stress or anxiety honestly, that being stressed is not your destiny. You learned that through the miracle of brain plasticity that you can rewrite your internal programing so that you feel more equanimity more of the time. You can rewire your brain to experience less anxiety while at the same time also experiencing more peace, more joy, more gratitude and appreciation, and a higher level of personal wellbeing.

You are separate from your stress; anxiety is not who you are, it is merely an emotion that you, that we all, experience from time to time during this human journey. Perhaps you can begin to view anxiety as it was intended to be viewed: As a loving protector that simply wants you to take control of the ship in order to assure the rest of the crew that everything is okay. Stress pops up to say, "Hey, would you mind addressing this? Those unnecessary thoughts are upsetting for me" or "Hello! Here I am! I don't like all of this negative social media…and by the way, we can find a better person to spend our time with!" Sometimes our anxiety can yell that there is a fire, when in all actuality there isn't even smoke, at which point you can choose to employ any of the tools and techniques that you have learned in order to calm your body and mind.

Hopefully you were able to try out the multiple mindful practices included in this guide and find something that works for you. Hopefully some of the mindful tips and free resources are also beneficial for you in your quest for overcoming stress and anxiety. Who would have known that just a yawn, a sigh, or a song could make such a world of difference? You now know that when you communicate to your body that it is safe through any myriad ways, including thinking authentically positive or happy thoughts, using humor or just consciously relaxing your muscles that your body will listen to you, and that it will respond accordingly.

You have the knowledge that simply having a positively-based faith can change your life for the better. The list of what you have read, and what you now know about overcoming and befriending stress and anxiety is vast. That is why education is the first half of your most powerful tool in this journey.

And awareness is the other half. Having an education doesn't get you very far if you do not use it. Self-awareness allows you to begin to unpack and recognize your own inner dialogue and personal belief system: You get the opportunity identify, meet, and know the real you, not the "you" that your stress tries to tell you that you are. When you are aware of the thoughts, events, people, locations and triggers that create anxiety for you then you can take the steps to mindfully change these situations, or at the very least, to mindfully change your reaction to these situations. When you are aware of the ways that stress presents itself in your body, you can sense it the moment it appears in order to address it quickly and efficiently – much like providing a coffee-to-go for a customer so that it can get the attention and service it needs and then happily move on.

In truth, the partnership of this knowledge and awareness isn't another tool for your toolbox, together they *are* the toolbox. All of the other tips, techniques, exercises, practices, and information are the tools that fit inside of this new container.

Know this: You are a magnificent, powerful being. The fact that you experience anxiety at times makes you human; perfectly human.

I hope you can feel the complete and utter sincerity in my words as I state that it is with everything in my heart that I wish you much love, health, happiness, joy, prosperity, awe, inspiration and peace in your life. You are an entirely empowered being with choice and control.

Let your bright light shine brightly.

**If you have found anything in these pages helpful or supportive for you, please consider spreading the word. With so much gratitude, Alex. **

Also by Alex Bruce

Breathe. Relax. Release: A Simple Guide to Meditation and Mindfulness

Finding Yourself Again: Making the Journey Back to You

Manufactured by Amazon.ca
Bolton, ON

31744987R00118